Food Fun with Trudy's ACTIVITY BOOK

by Norma McCormick

ISBN : 978-1-7373058-1-1

Published by Harmony ‘n Abundance LLC
www.gertieslivinggardens.com
Graphic Design : RachelKarpf@outlook.com

PUZZLE TIME

Food Crossword

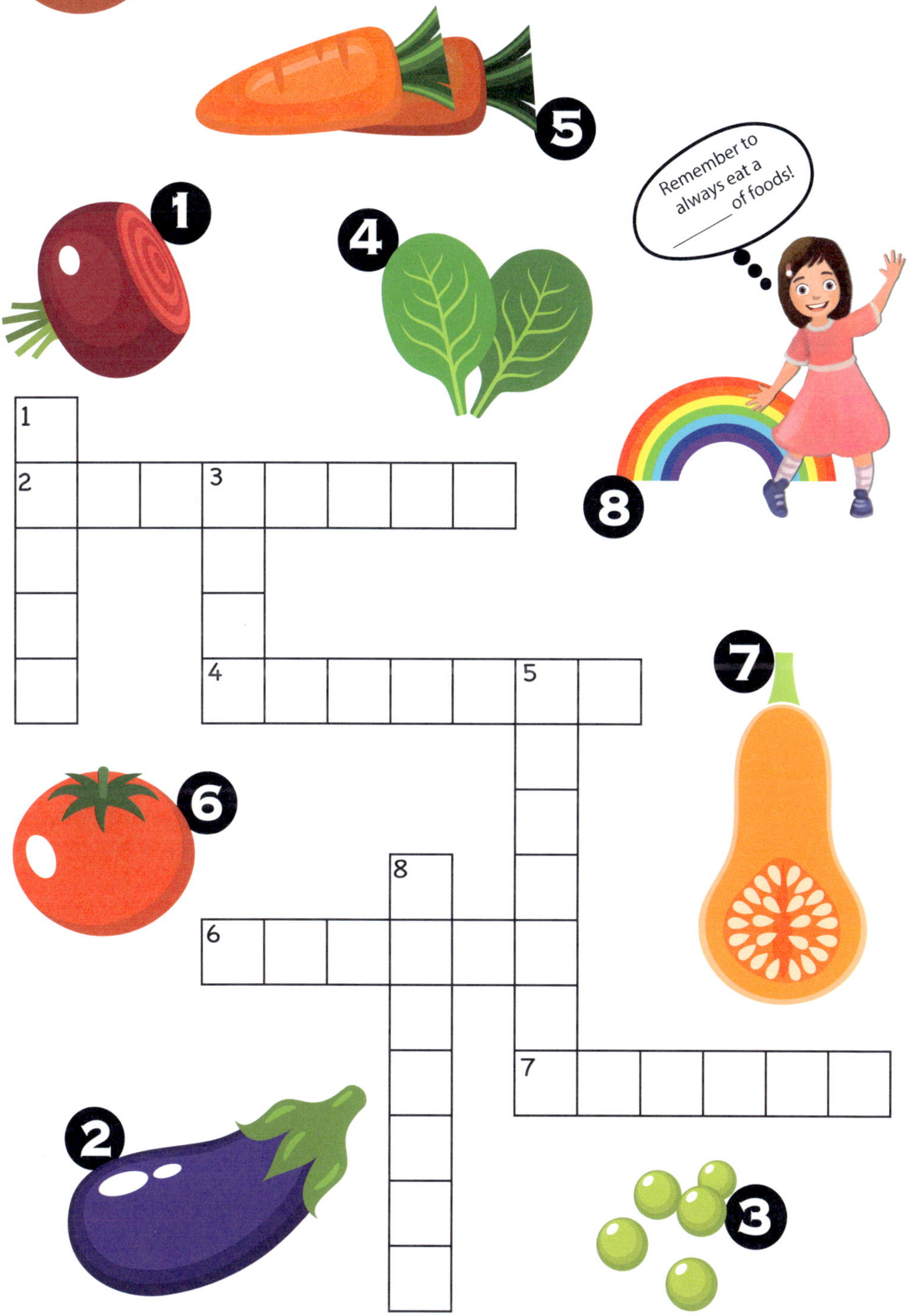

PUZZLE TIME

Connect the Dots

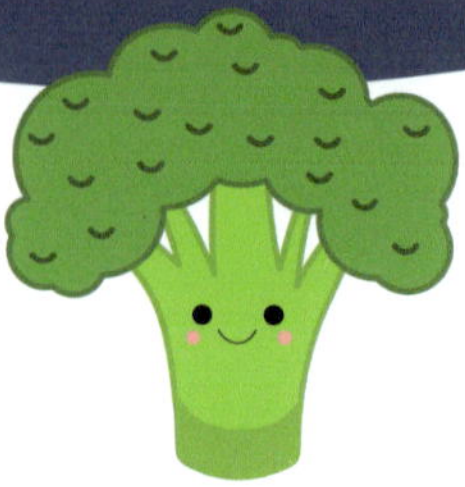

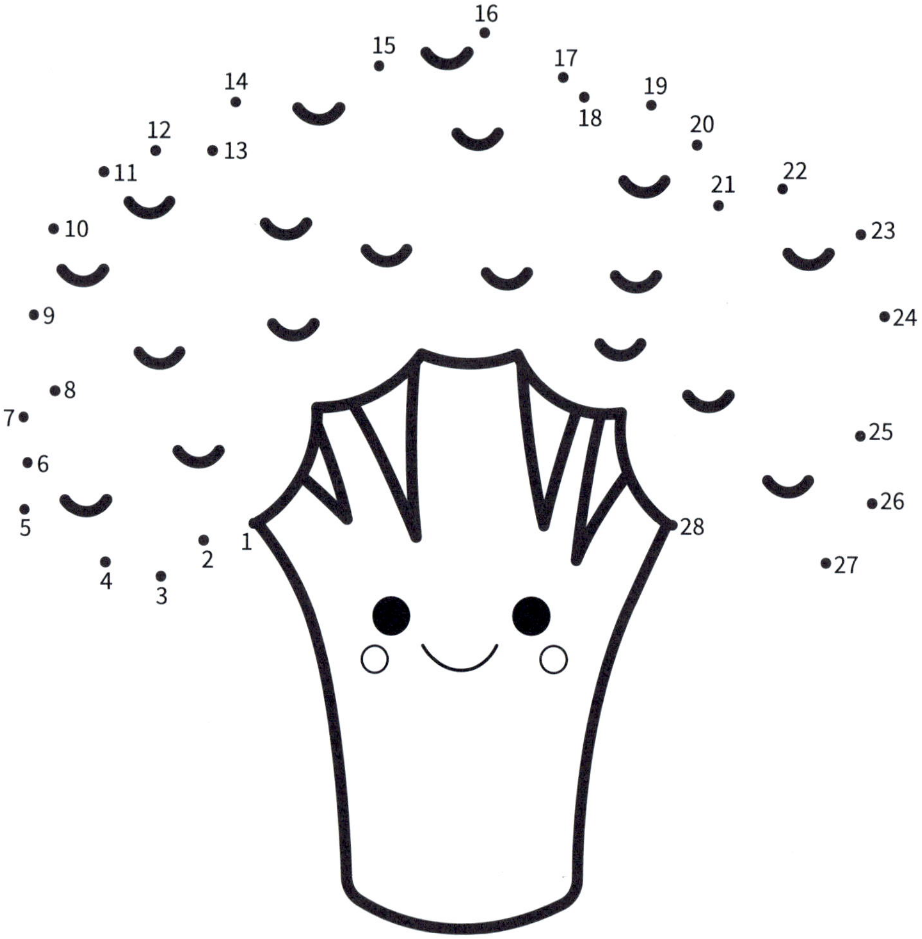

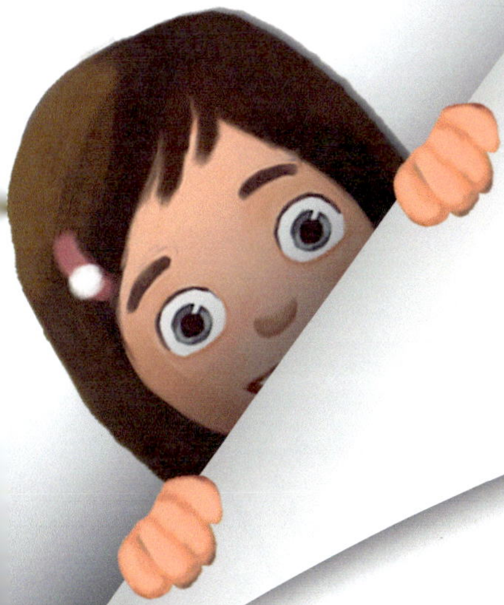

Did you know?

You can Build your Own Garden!

1. Find an area in your yard that is suitable for you.

2. Ensure it gets a lot of sunlight, has the best soil and is near a water source.

3. Choose the layout for your vegetable garden. It does not necessarily have to be the usual rectangular shape.

4. The soil you have in your yard may be used for your garden. Make sure though it is free of weeds and insects which can harm seedlings.

5. Choose the right kinds of vegetables to plant. Find the list of vegetables that are easy to grow.

6. Have fun and watch your veggies grow!

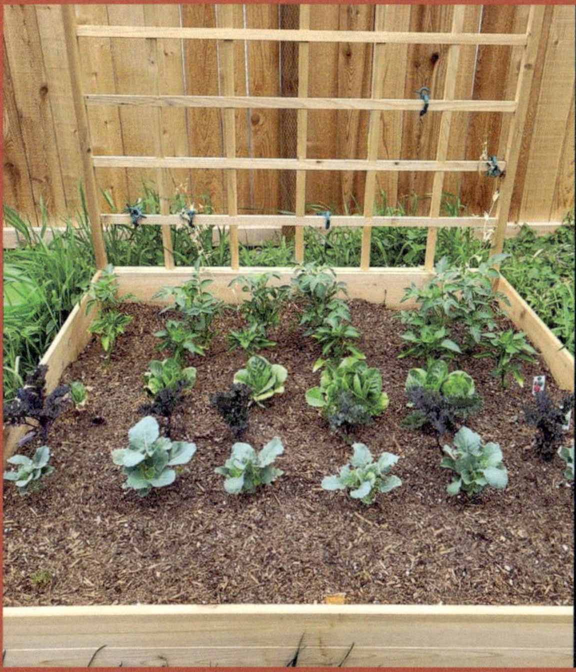

Tomatoes
Cherry tomatoes
Radish
Broccoli
Carrots
Cucumber
Cabbage
Beets
Beans
Peas
Strawberries
Eggplants
Squash

ART TIME

Let's Color

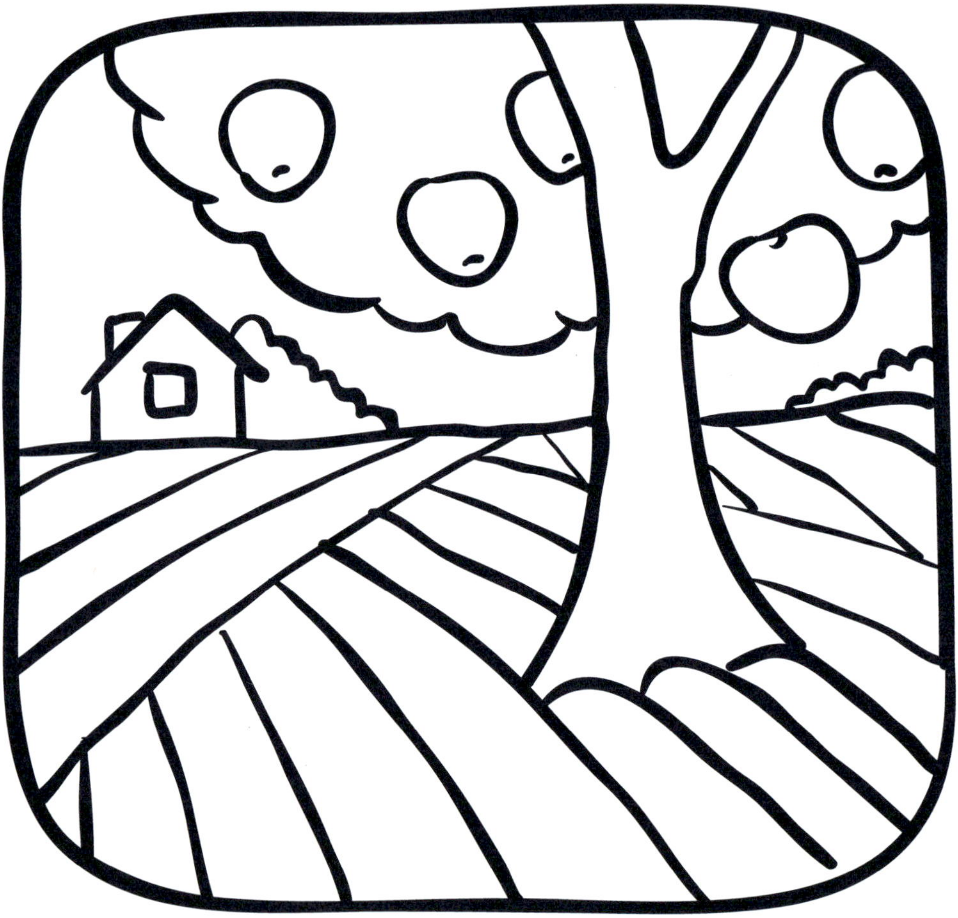

QUIZ TIME

What Food Group is it?

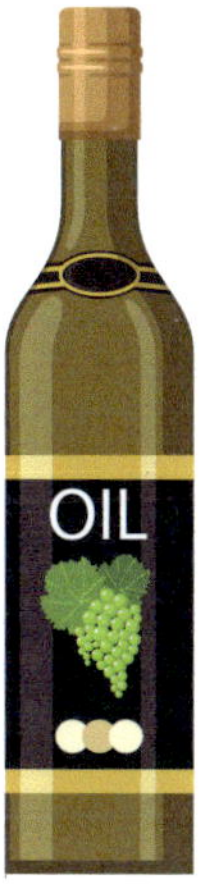

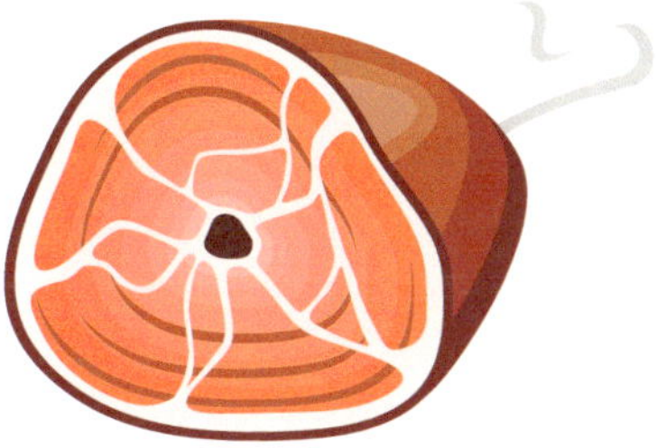

CARB

FAT

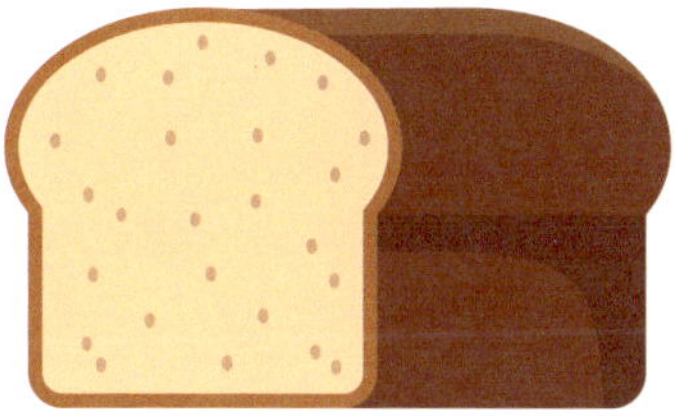

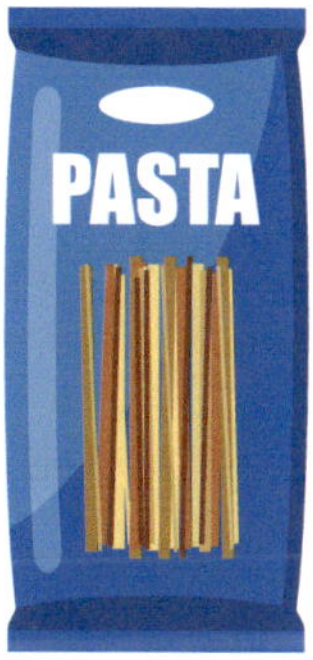

PROTEIN

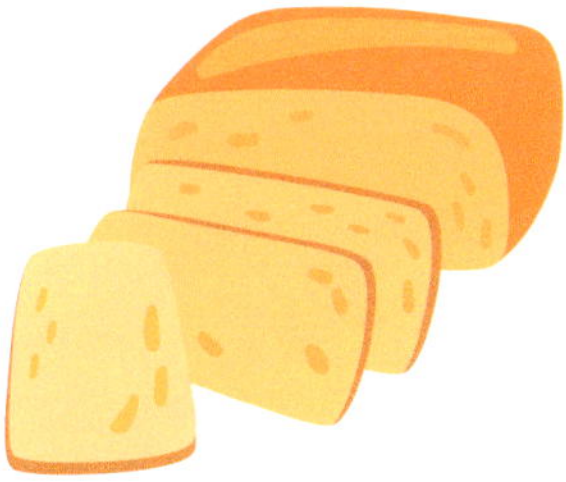

FIBER

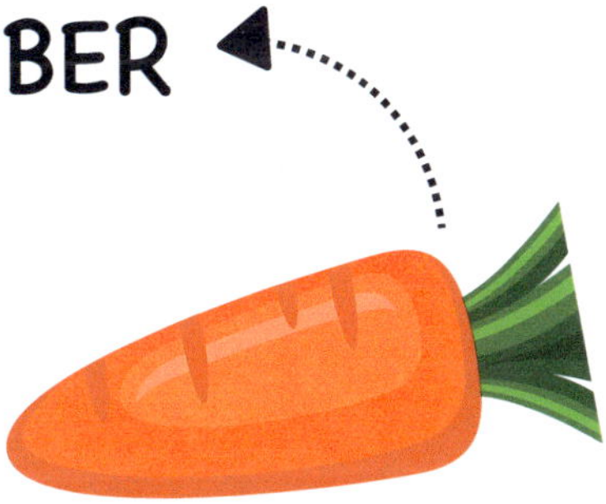

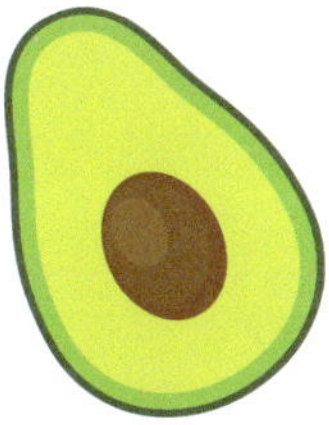

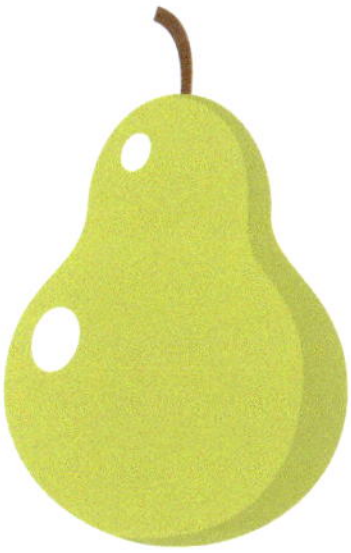

PUZZLE TIME

Help the Pumpkin Escape

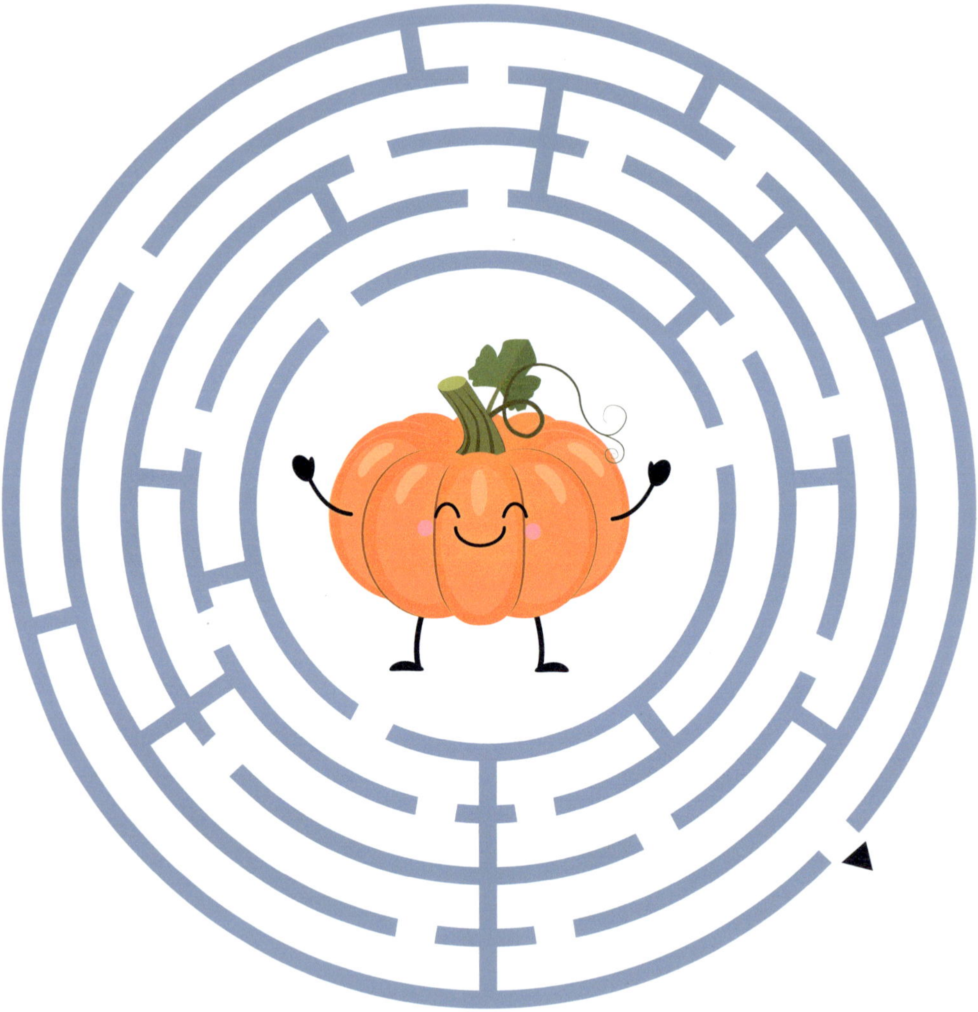

QUIZ TIME

Match Tops to the Bottoms

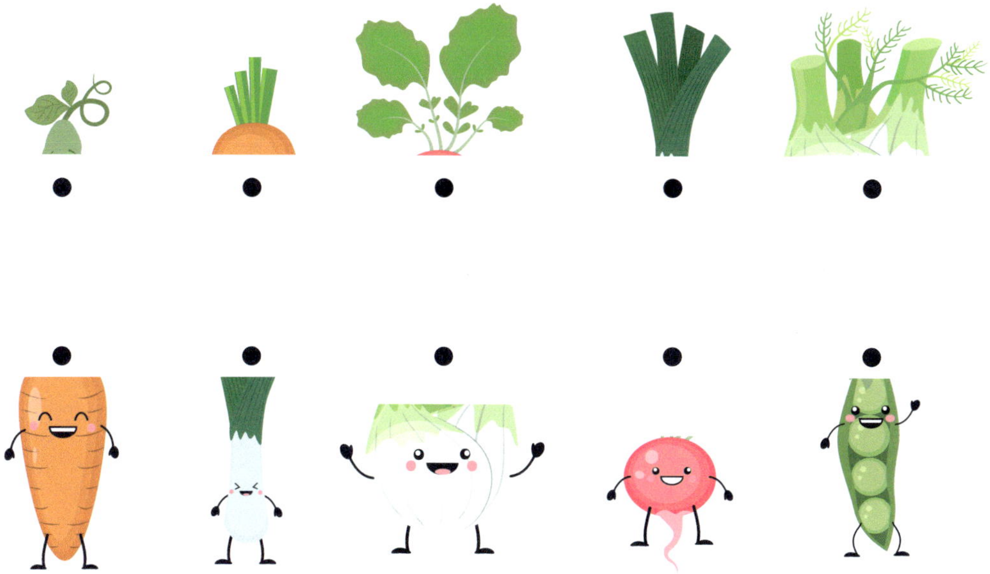

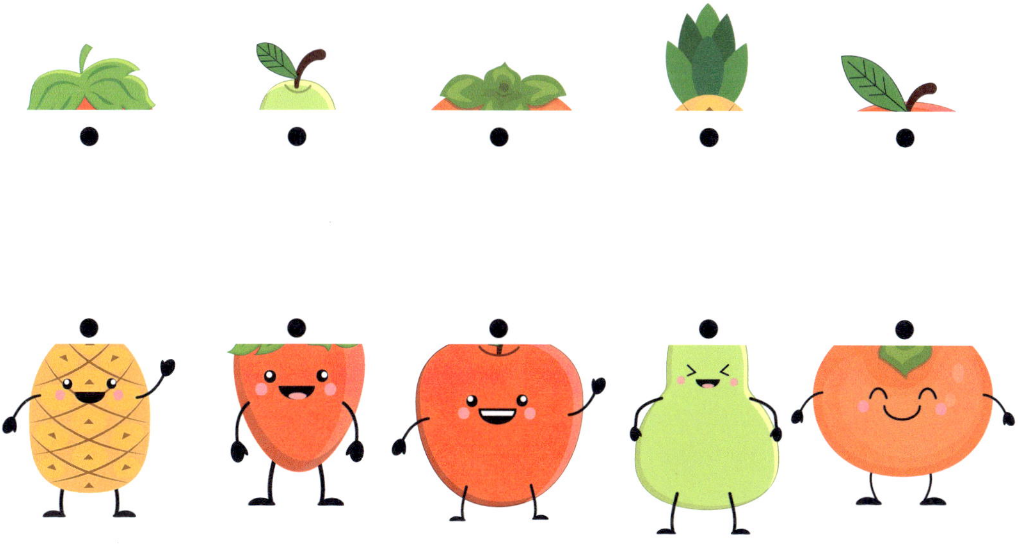

QUIZ TIME

Count How Many

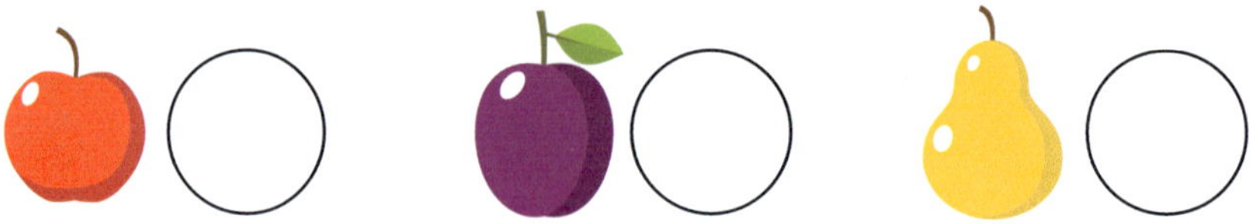

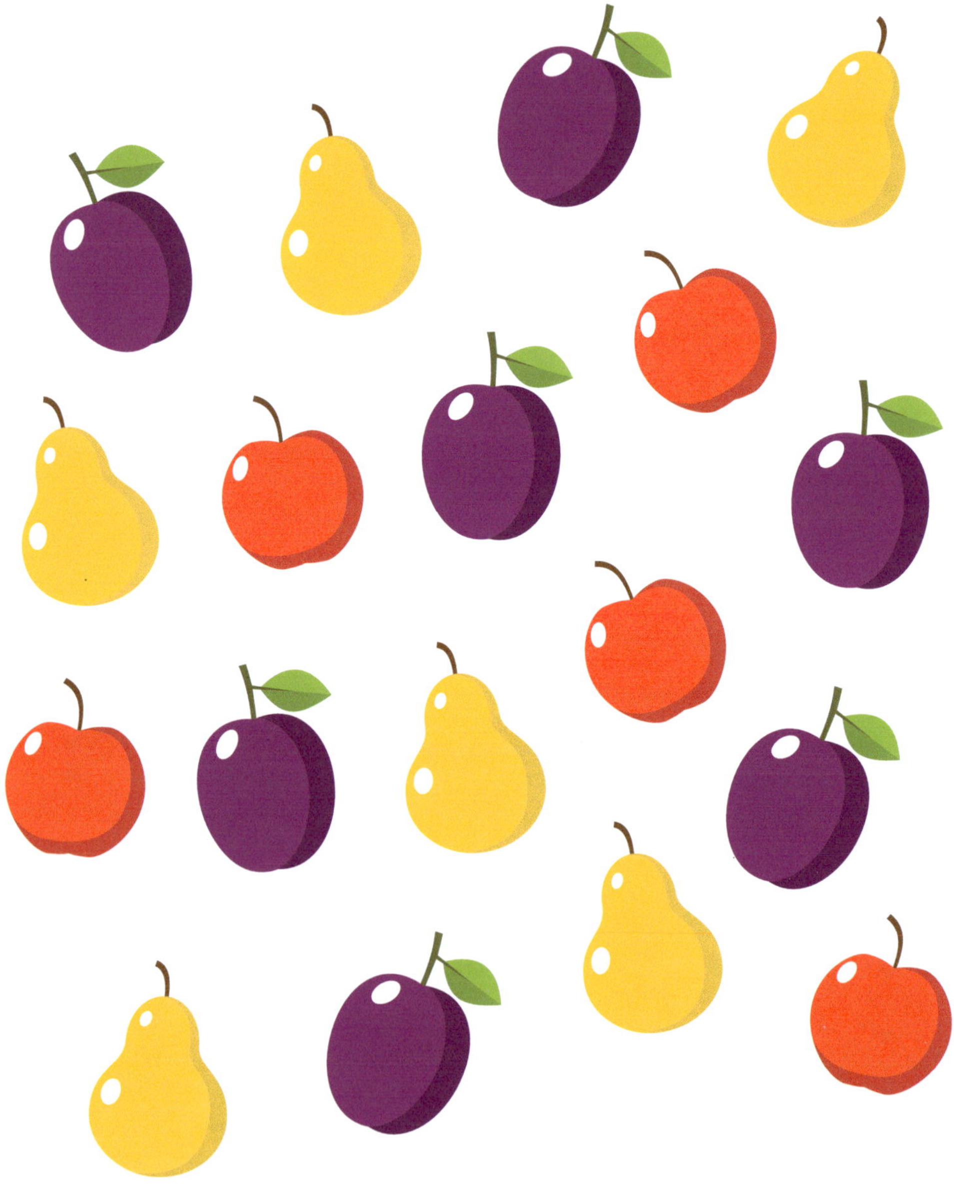

PUZZLE TIME

Fruit Word Search

L	O	H	P	E	A	C	H	K	C
I	R	A	P	P	L	E	N	O	O
P	A	B	A	N	A	N	A	C	C
L	N	S	O	N	D	A	M	J	O
U	G	Y	G	R	A	P	E	S	N
M	E	A	E	M	O	G	N	I	U
P	I	N	E	A	P	P	L	E	T
S	E	L	M	Y	K	L	O	I	D
P	A	P	E	A	R	M	E	R	S
W	Y	Z	O	R	L	E	M	O	N

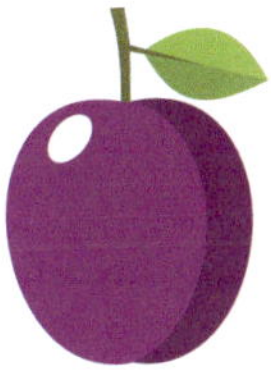

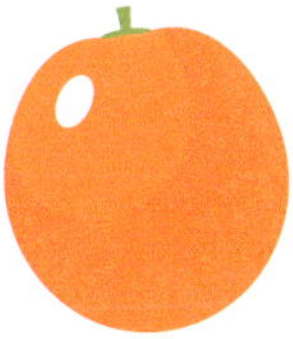
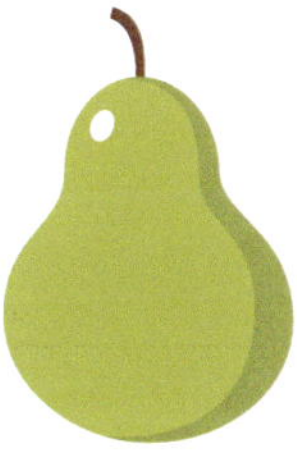

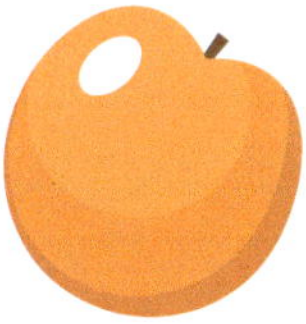
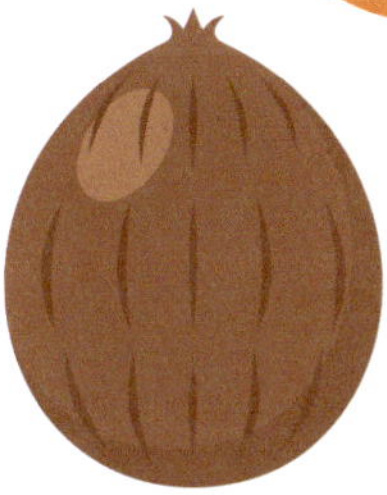

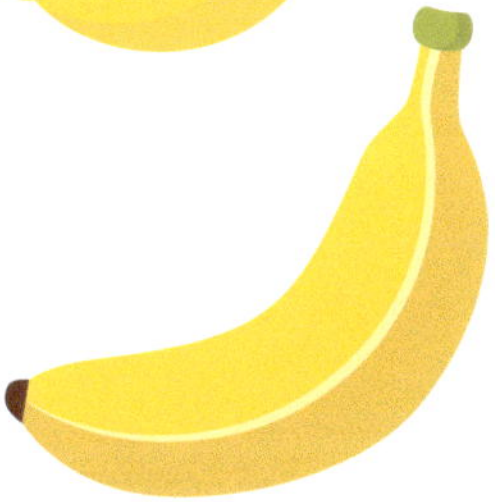

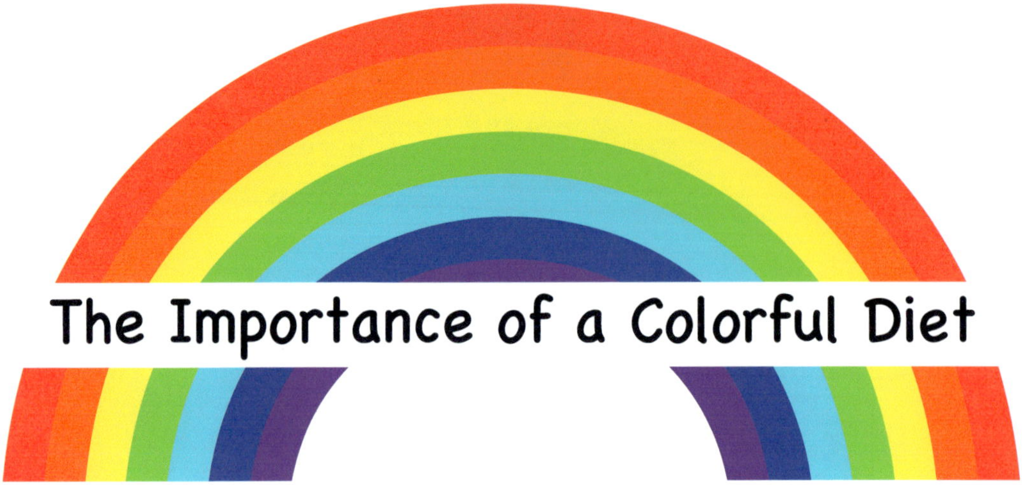

The Importance of a Colorful Diet

Red Fruits and Vegetables- protect our hearts and improve brain function. Most red fruits and vegetables contain antioxidants to keep us healthy.

Red Vegetables: tomatoes, radishes, red cabbage, beets

Red Fruits: red grapes, strawberries, watermelon, cherries, raspberries, pomegranates, cranberries, and red apples

Blue and Purple Fruits and Vegetables- help prevent heart disease, stroke and cancer. Blue and purple fruits and vegetables are important for memory, promote healthy aging and regulate healthy digestion.

Blue and Purple Vegetables: eggplant, purple cabbage, purple potatoes

Blue and Purple Fruits: blackberries, blueberries, purple grapes, plums, raisins, figs

Orange and Yellow Fruits and Vegetables- are packed with nutrients that are known to protect your nervous system promote eye health and prevent heart diseases. They also play an important role in maintaining skin health, boosting your immune system and helping build strong bones.

Orange and Yellow Vegetables: carrots, pumpkin, sweet corn, sweet potato, yellow pepper, yellow tomatoes

Orange and Yellow Fruits: yellow apples, apricots, oranges, grapefruit, peaches, mangoes, papaya, pears, pineapple

Green fruits and vegetables- Green fruits and vegetables protect eye health. Essential nutrients found in green fruits and vegetables help regulate digestion and improve immune system functioning.

Green Vegetables: broccoli, spinach, cabbage, lettuce, Brussels sprouts, green beans, cucumbers, zucchini, peas, green pepper

Green Fruits: green apples, kiwi, green grapes, lime, avocado

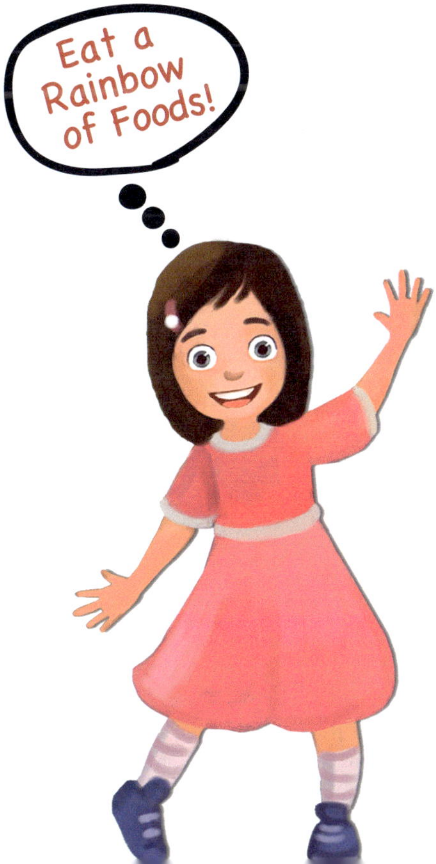

ART TIME

Complete the Picture

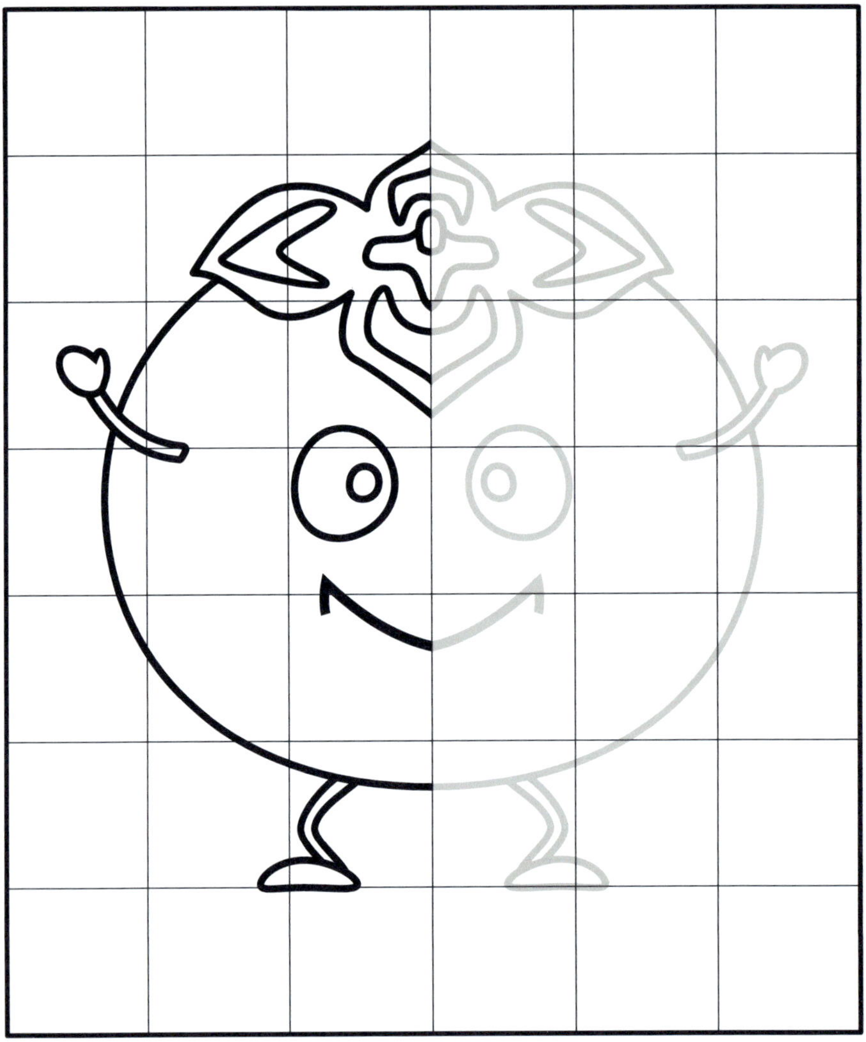

JOKE TIME

Knock Knock Jokes

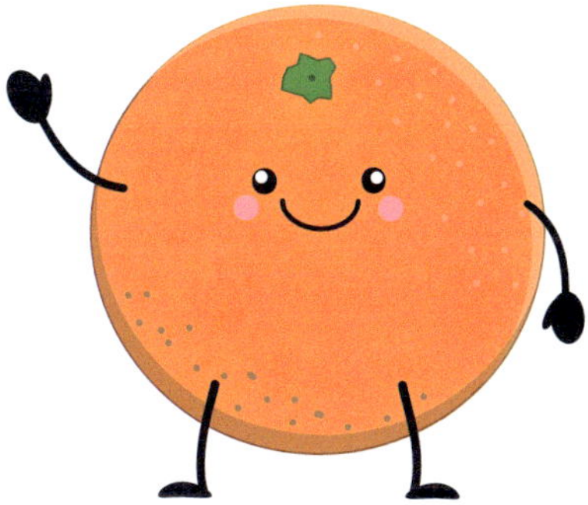

Knock Knock
Who's there?!
Banana!
Banana who?
Banana split so ice creamed!

Knock Knock
Who's there?
Orange
Orange who?
Orange you going to answer the door?

Knock Knock
Who's there?
Lettuce
Lettuce who?
Lettuce go before you eat me!

Knock Knock
Who's there?
Turnip
Turnip who?
Turnip the volume, it's my favorite song!

Knock Knock
Who's there?
Leaf!
Leaf who?
Leaf me alone.

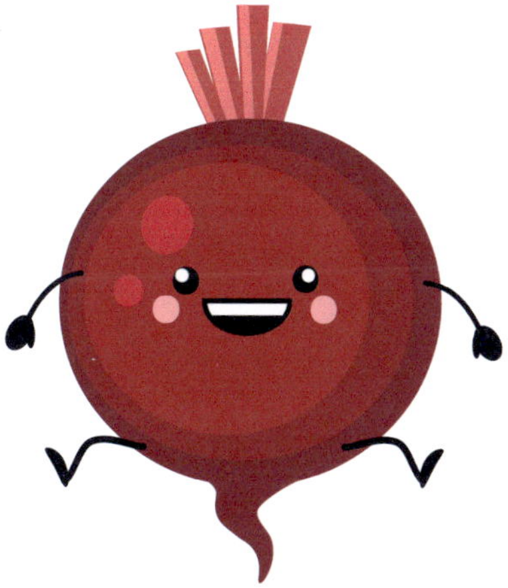

Knock Knock
Who's there?
Egg!
Egg who?
Egg-celent question!

Knock Knock
Who's there?
Olive!
Olive who?
Olive you!

ART TIME

Let's Color

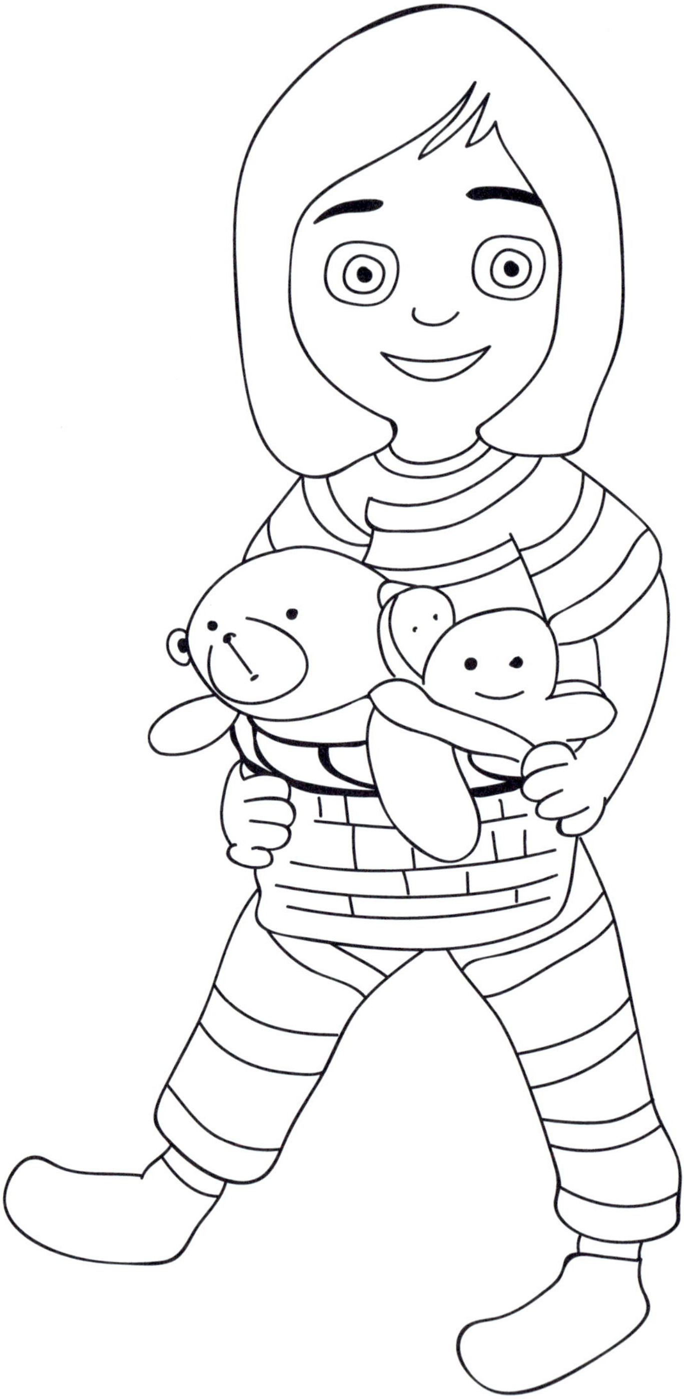

ART TIME

Complete the Picture

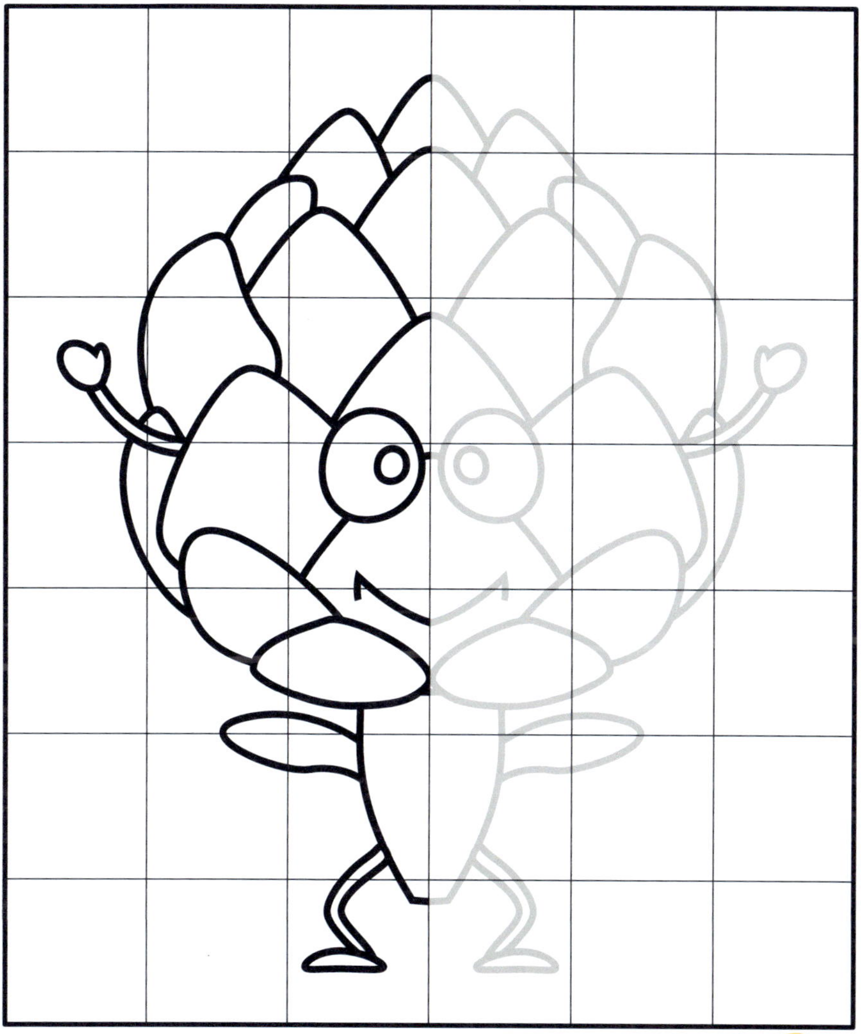

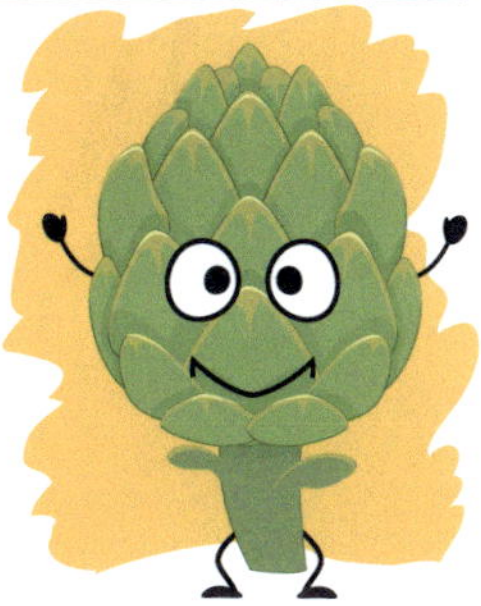

ART TIME

Let's Color

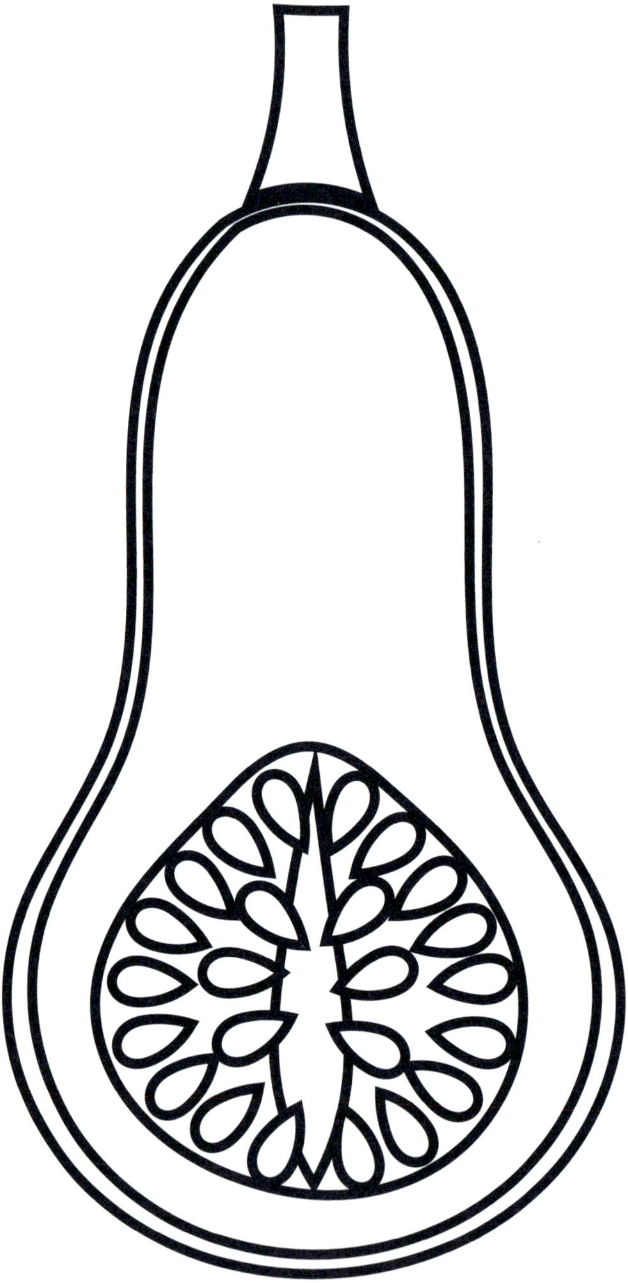

ART TIME

Paper Dolls

Making a chain of paper dolls is a classic paper craft. It's fun, easy, and may become a tradition in your family. This project require scissors so adult supervision is recommended.

1. Take a piece of paper (8.5" x 11") and cut it lengthwise.

2. Fold it into quarters accordion (pleated) style.

3. Draw a figure of a person on the top layer. Be sure that the arms extend beyond the edge of the folded sheet. You can draw your own figure or use the templates below.

4. Cut the figure out and unfold. You will get a chain of dolls holding hands.

5. To have more dolls in your chain, use a larger sheet of paper and fold more pleats before cutting. Alternatively, use more than one sheet of paper and connect the figures with tape.

6. You can decorate the figures with eyes, nose, mouth, hair, and clothes. You can make variations such as paper figures that wear dresses (women), look like teddy bears, or like ginger bread men.

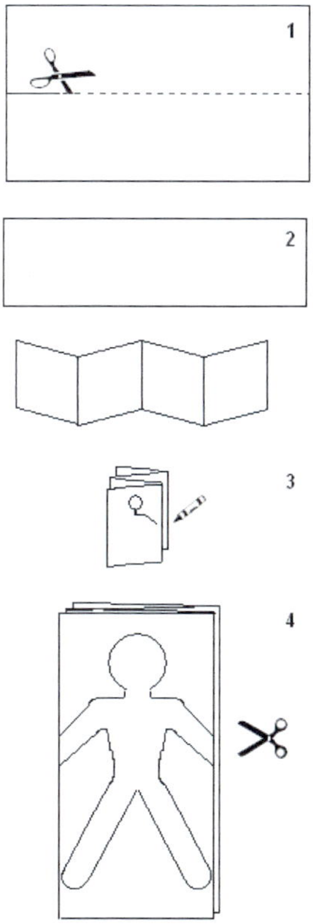

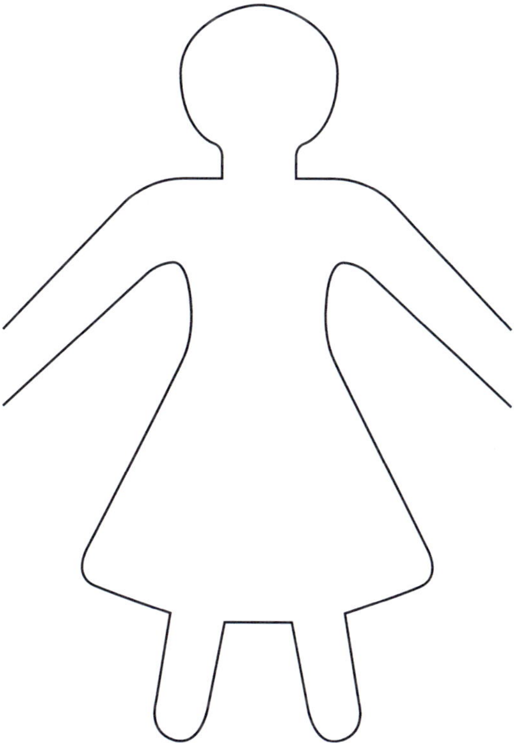

PUZZLE TIME

Find the Correct Shape

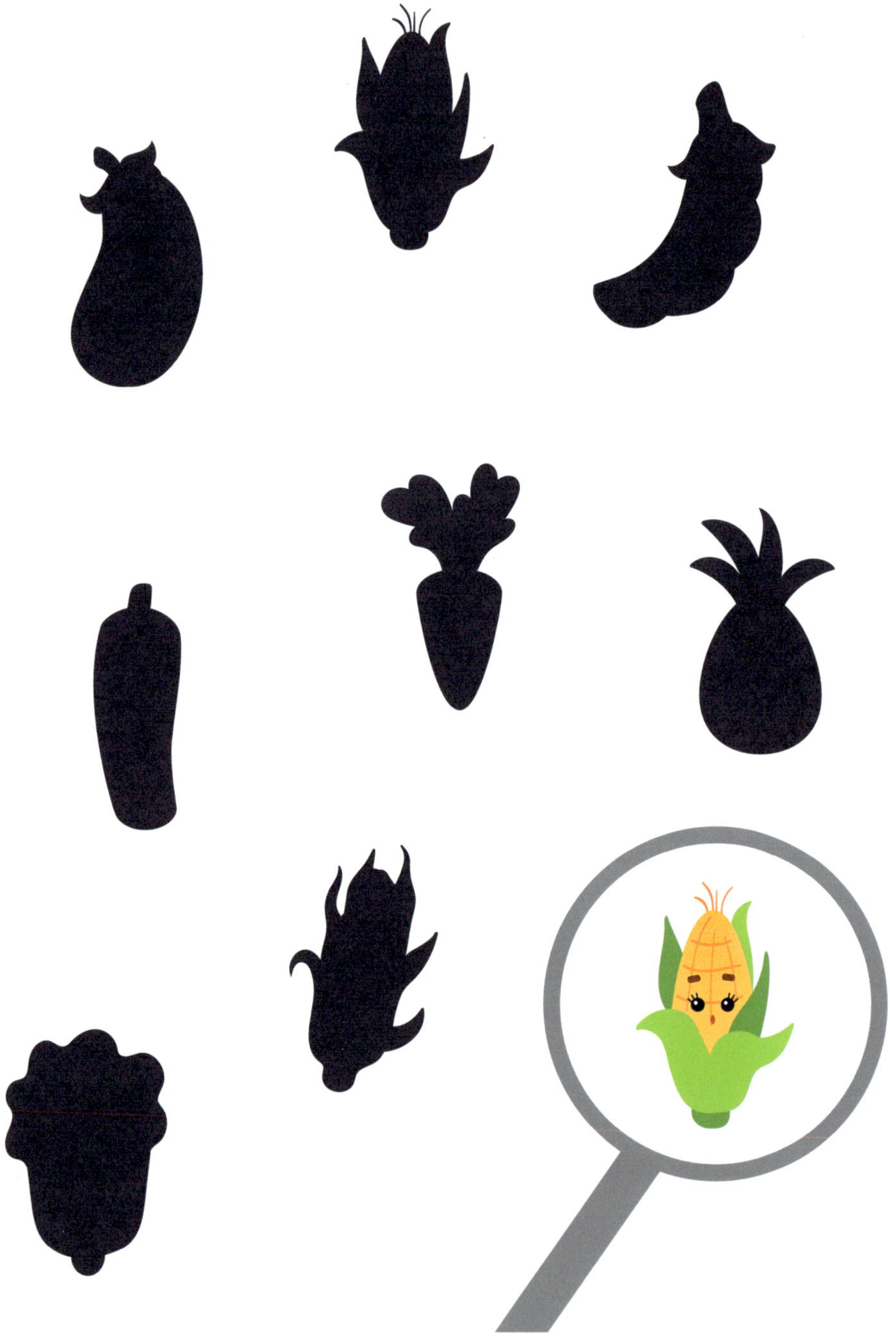

PUZZLE TIME

Connect the Dots

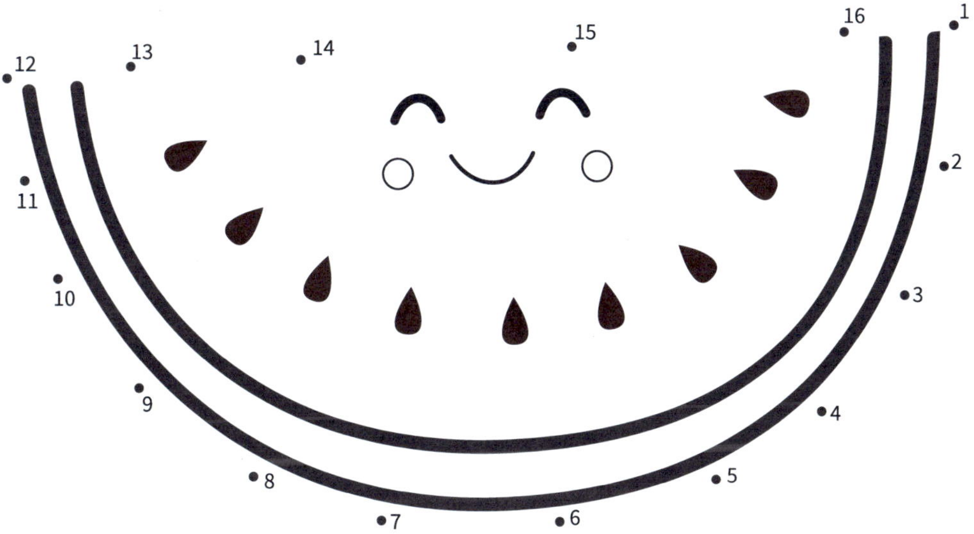

ART TIME

Let's Color

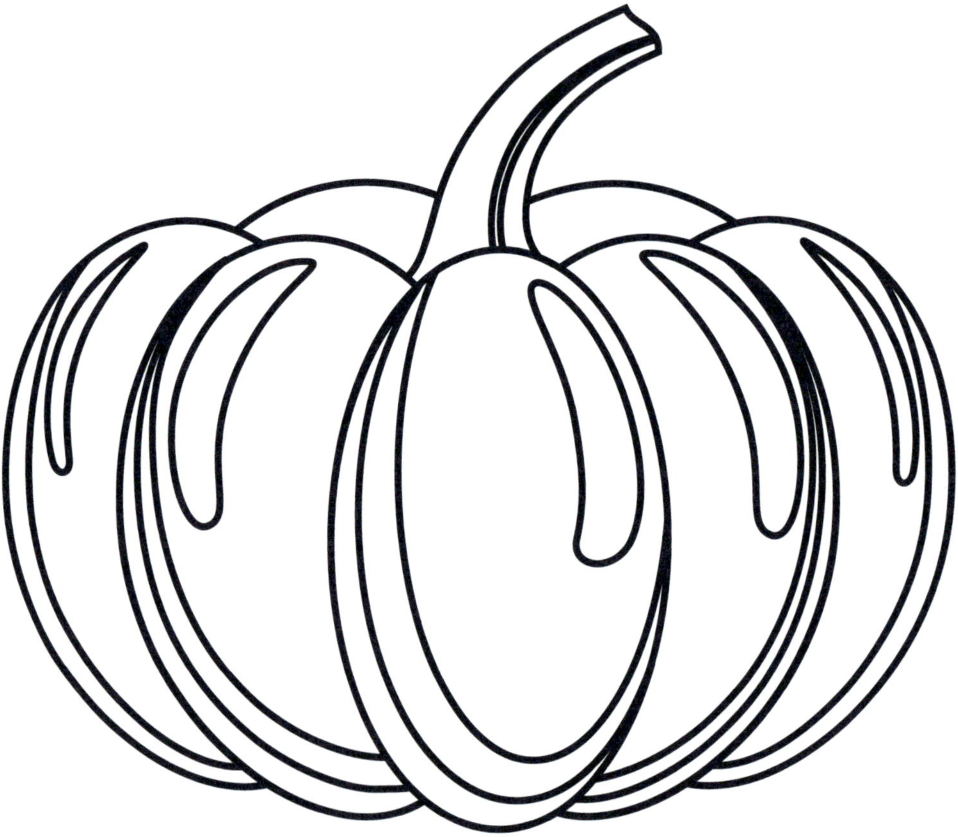

Did you know?

A fruit develops from the flower of a plant, while the other parts of the plant are categorized as vegetables. Fruits contain seeds, while vegetables can consist of roots, stems and leaves.

Are Bananas a vegetable? Yes, they are. They are a tropical fruit crop grown by millions of people all over the world, and have long been an integral part of the cultural diet. The most commonly seen fruits are the yellow, green, and black bananas, but it is the banana that get the most attention.

Sweet potatoes are nutrient-dense root vegetables that come in a variety of colors. They're high in fiber and antioxidants, which protect your body from free radical damage and promote a healthy gut and brain.

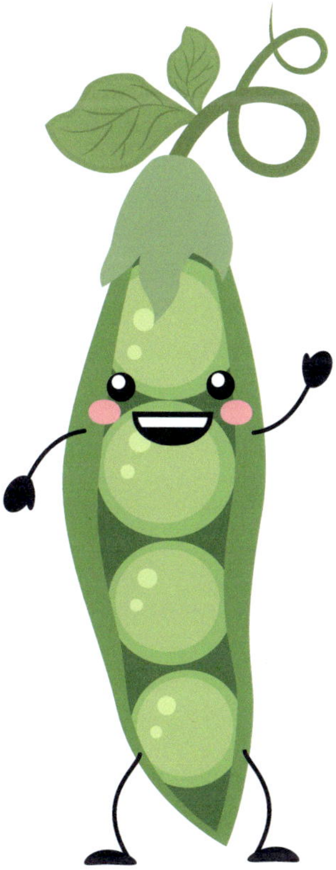

Most berries grow on bushes, which can be neat shrubs like cultivated raspberries and gooseberries to dense, spiky thickets like wild blackberries. Apples are incredibly good for you, and eating them is linked to a lower risk of many major diseases, including diabetes and cancer. What's more, its soluble fiber content may promote weight loss and gut health. A medium apple equals 1.5 cups of fruit — which is 3/4 of the 2-cup daily recommendation for fruit.

PUZZLE TIME

Match the Fruits & Vegetables

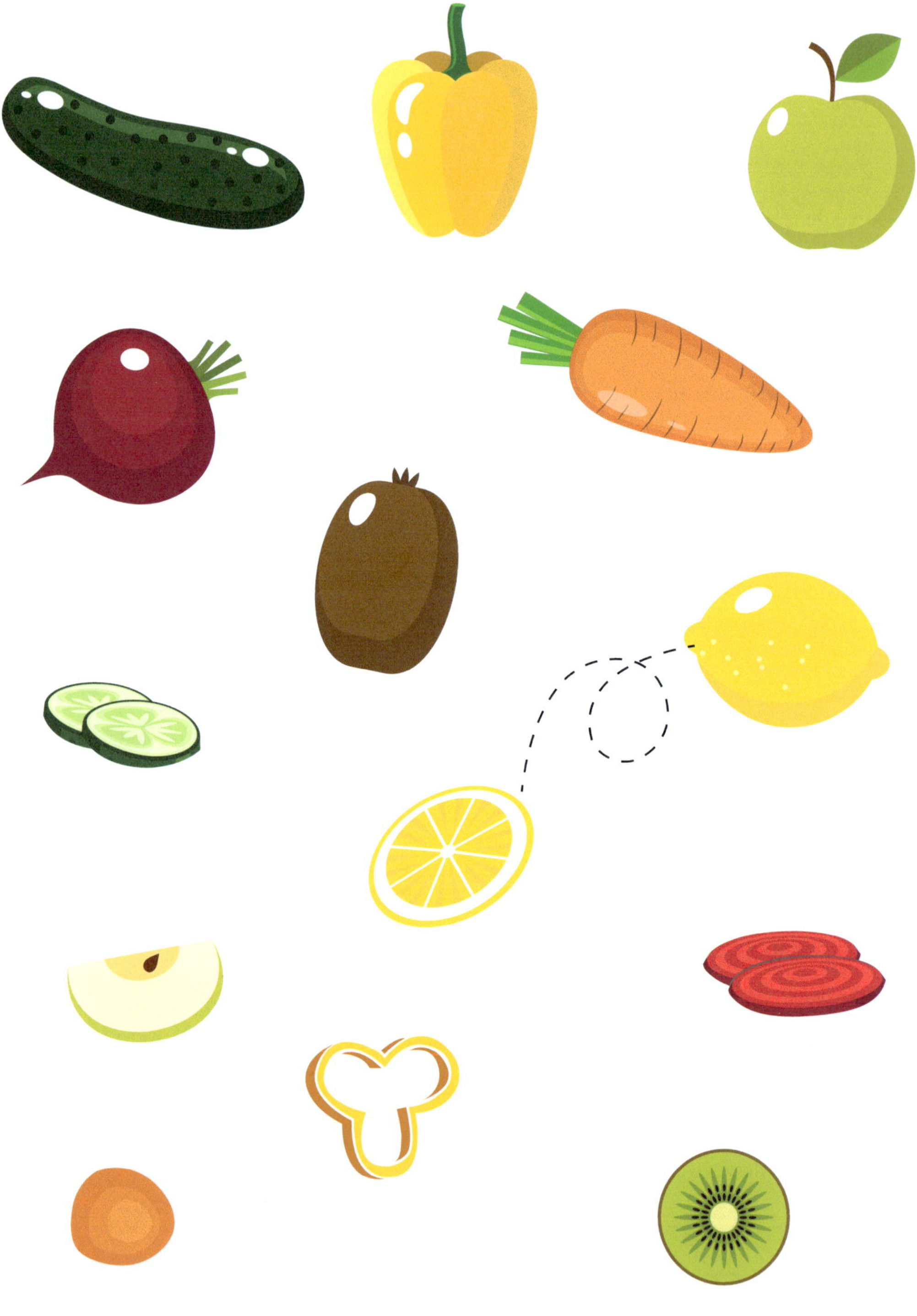

PUZZLE TIME

Fruit Crossword

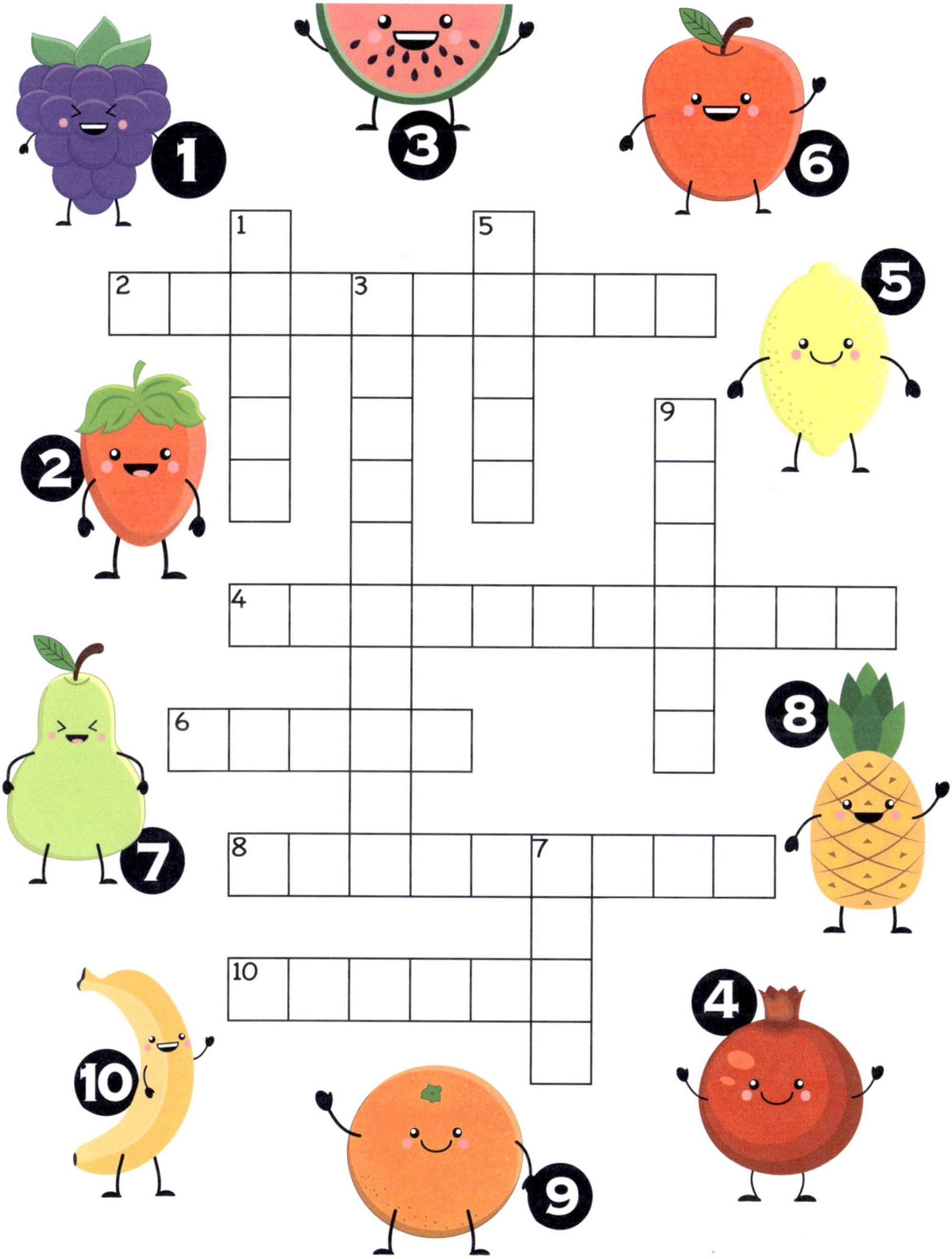

ART TIME

Color Your Favorite Activities

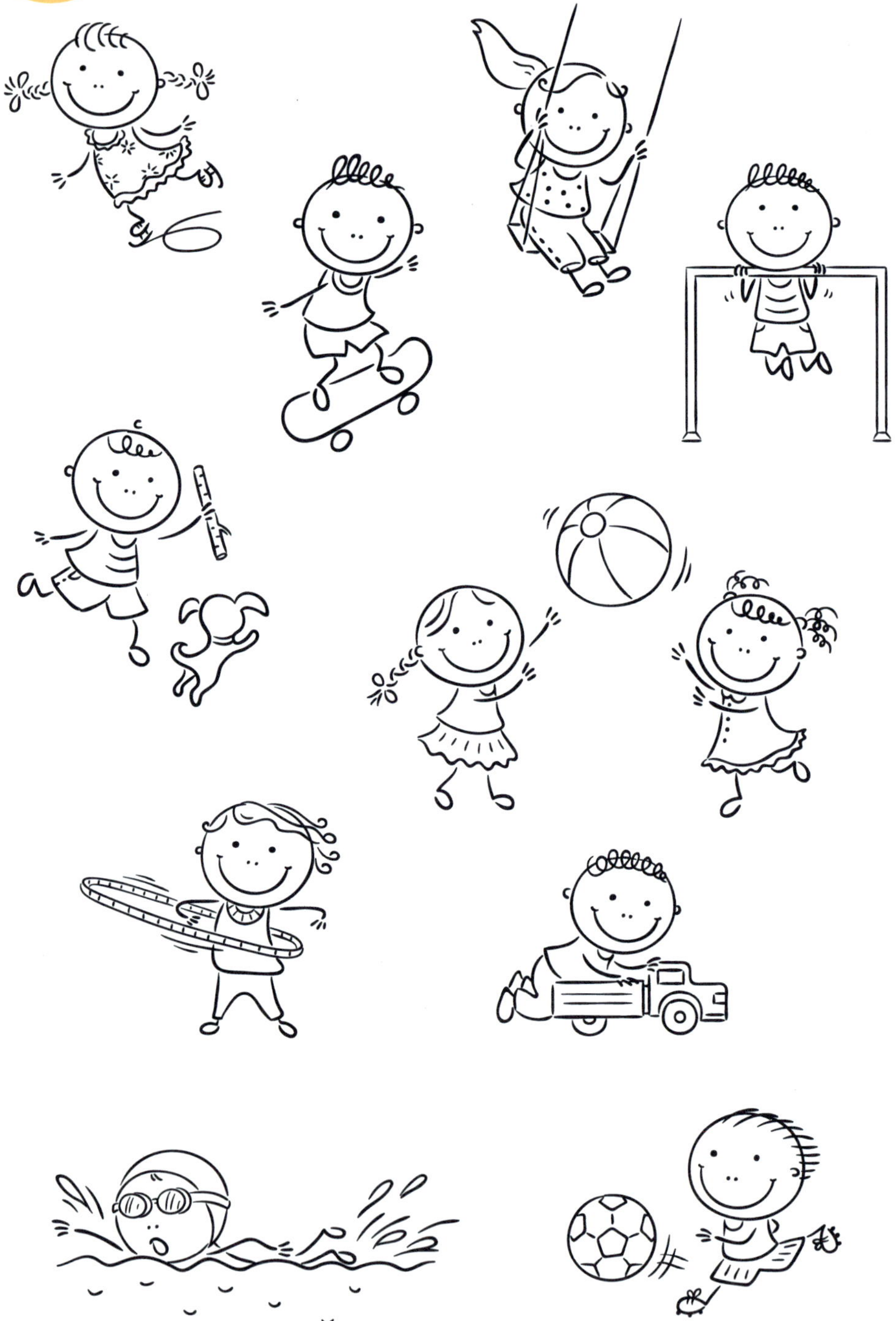

PUZZLE TIME

Help Orange Find His Way

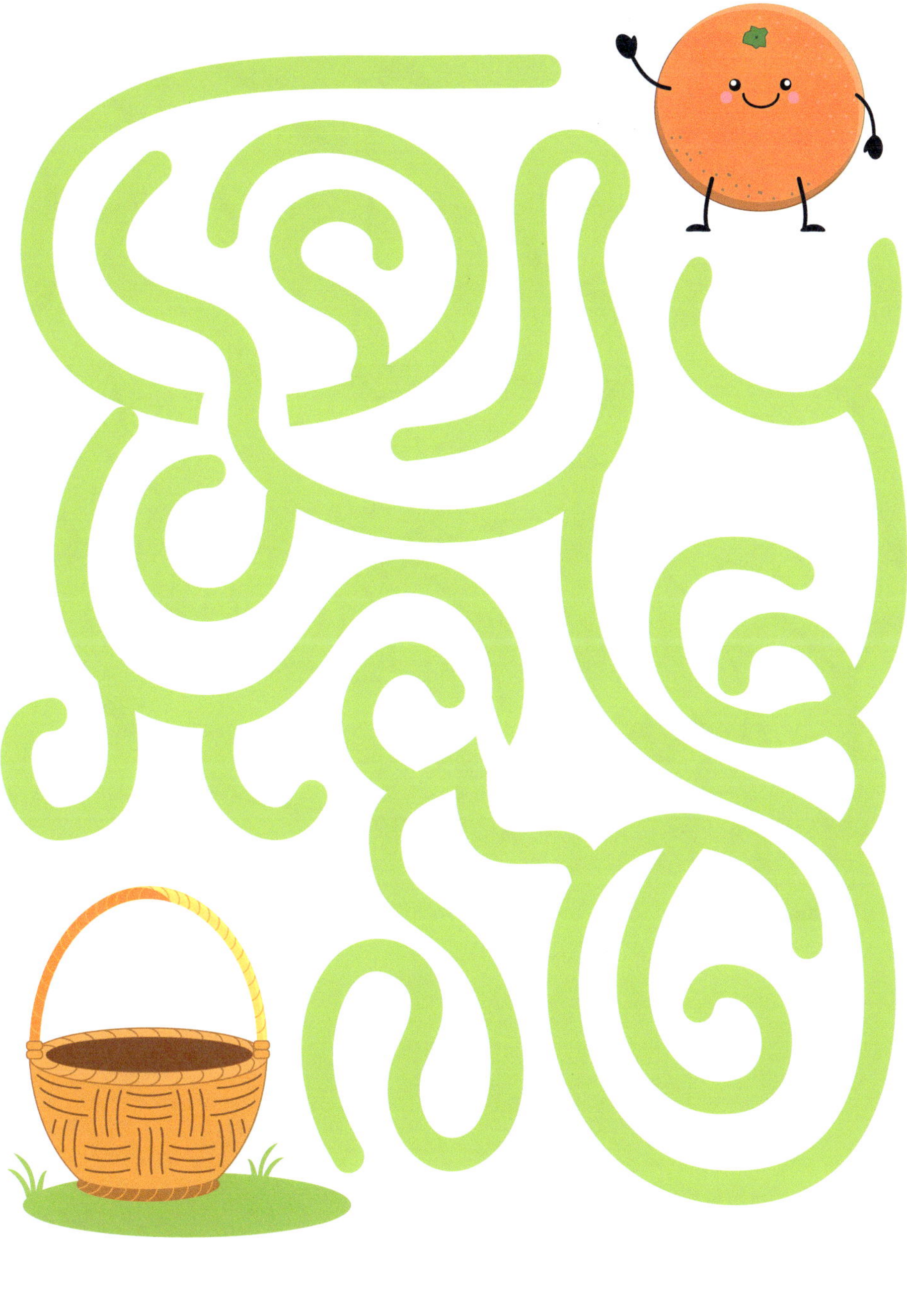

ART TIME

Let's Color

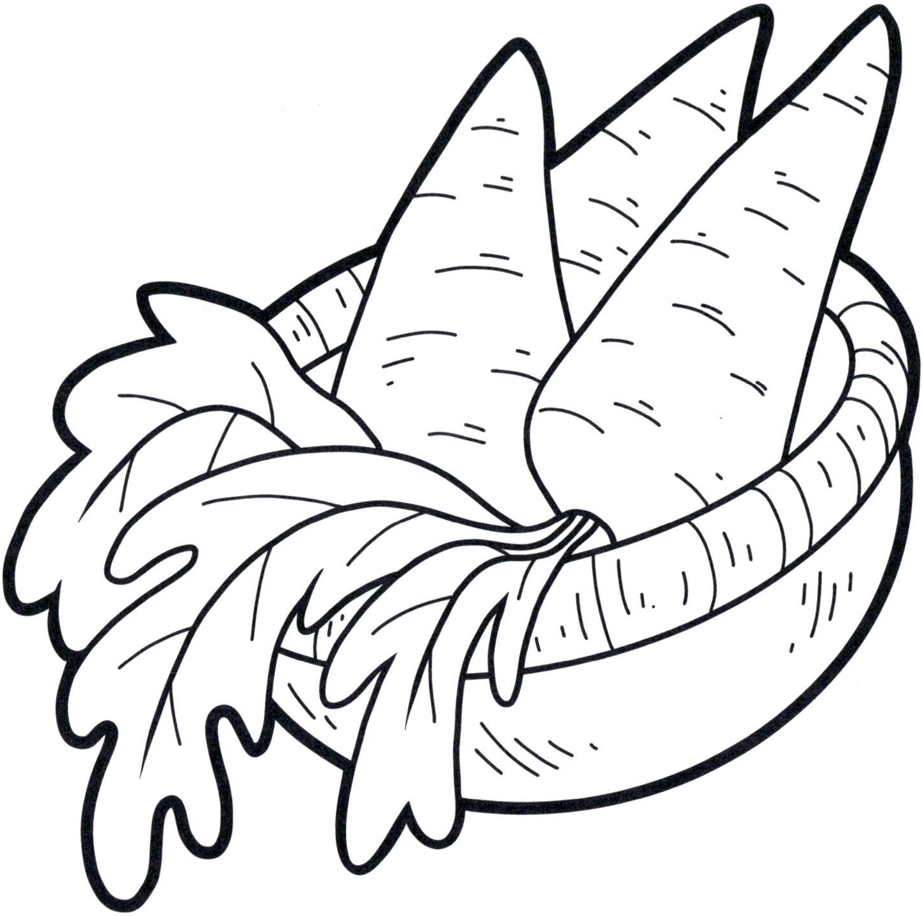

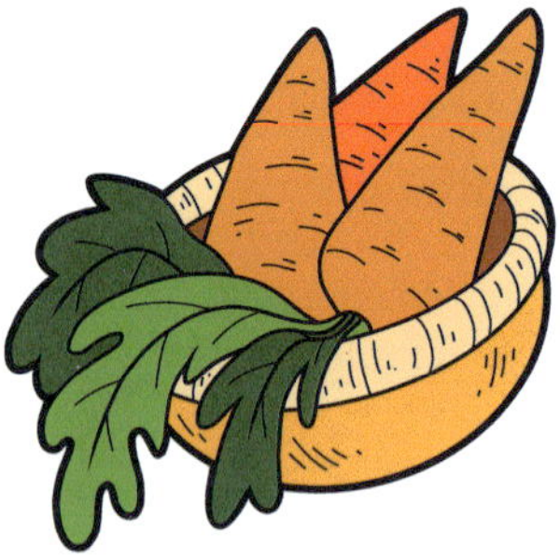

TRIVIA TIME

Put the Pictures in Order

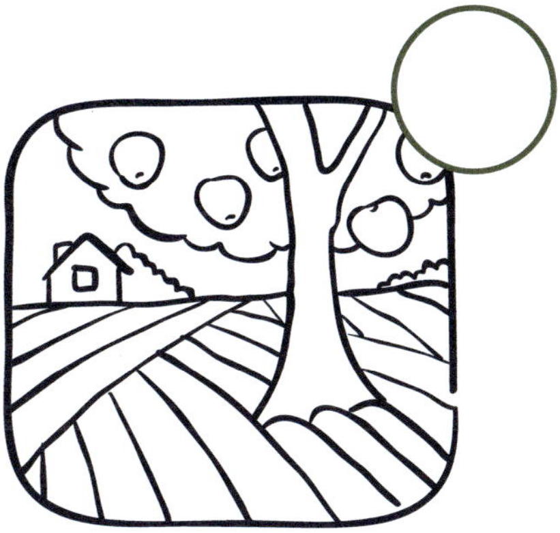

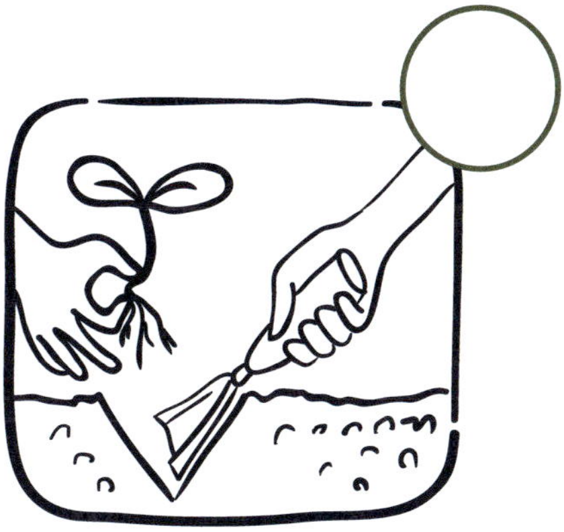

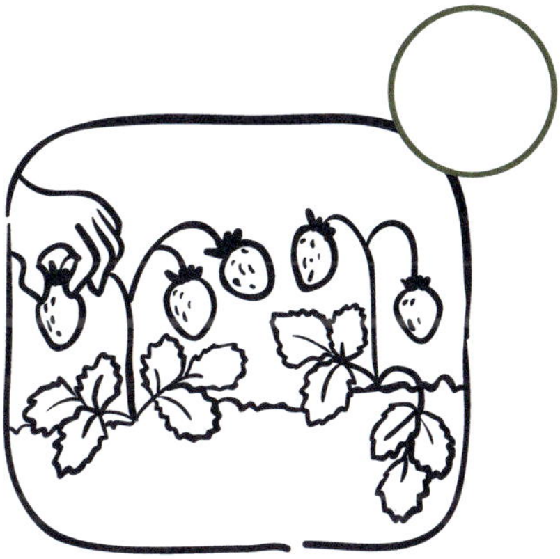

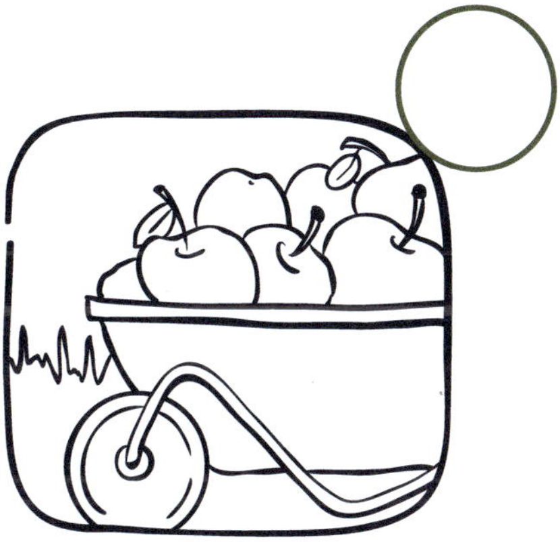

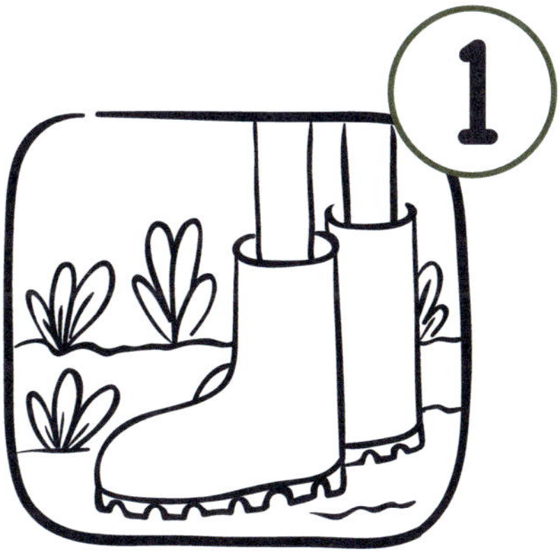

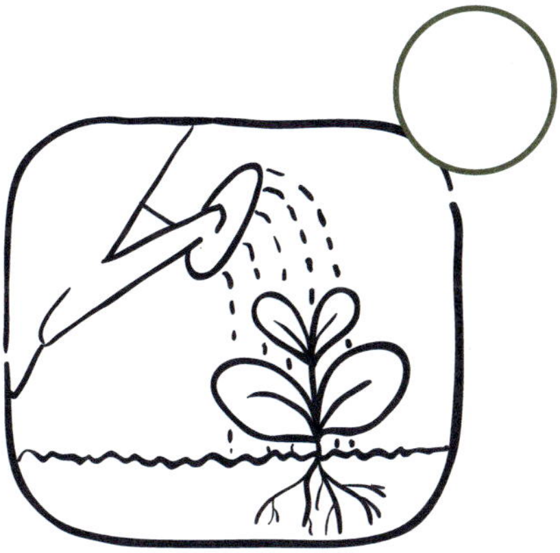

Let's Color

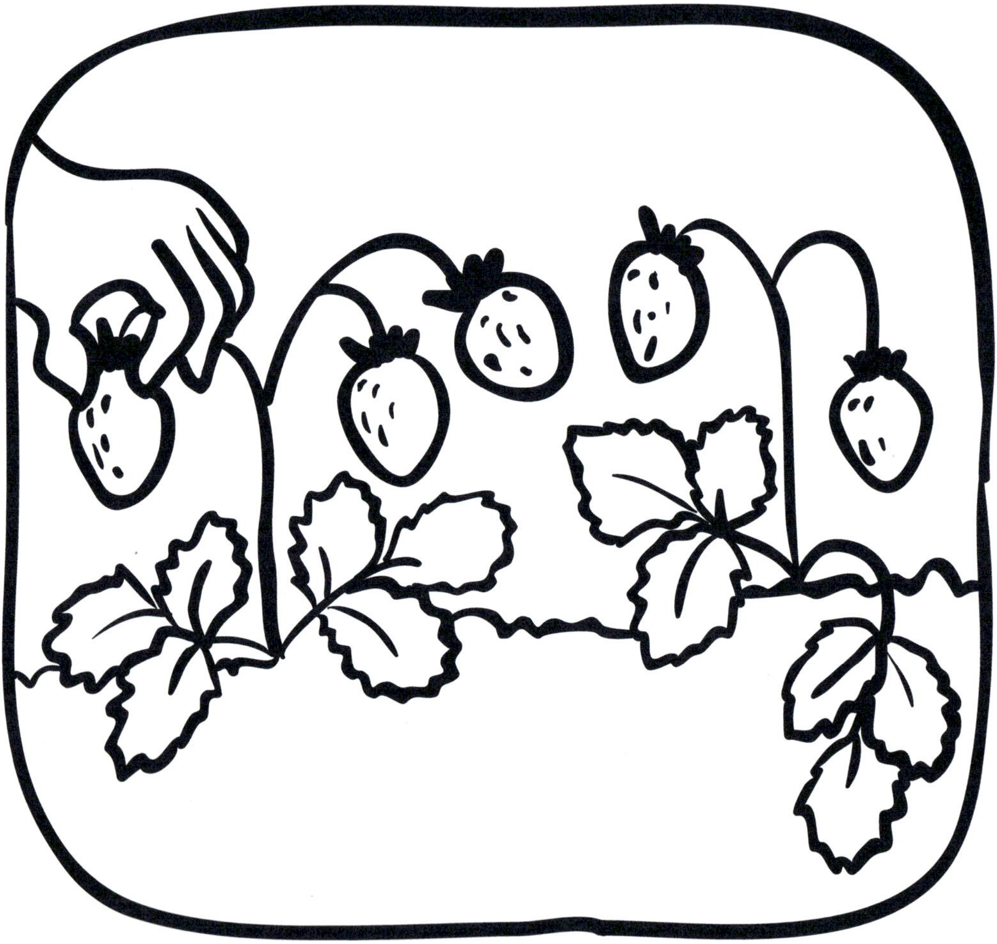

ART TIME

Let's Color

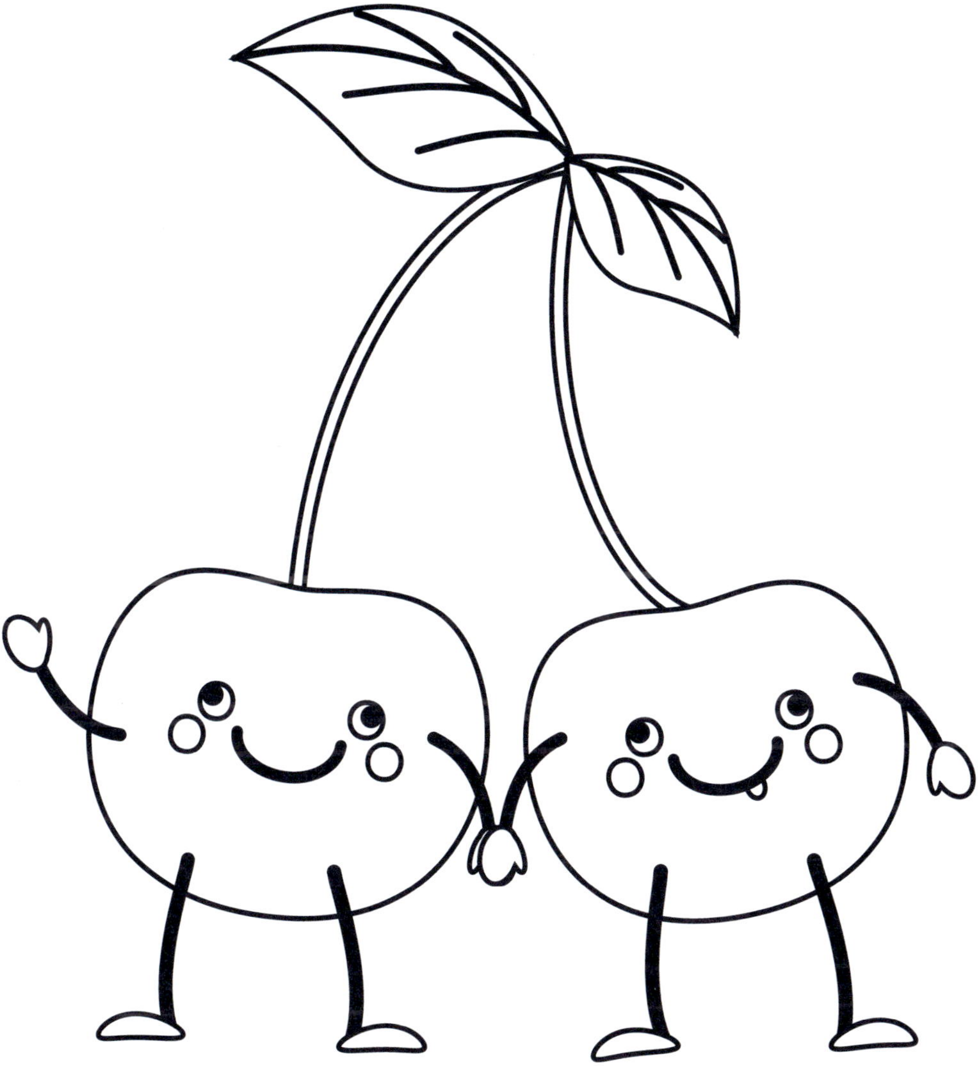

Find the 10 Differences

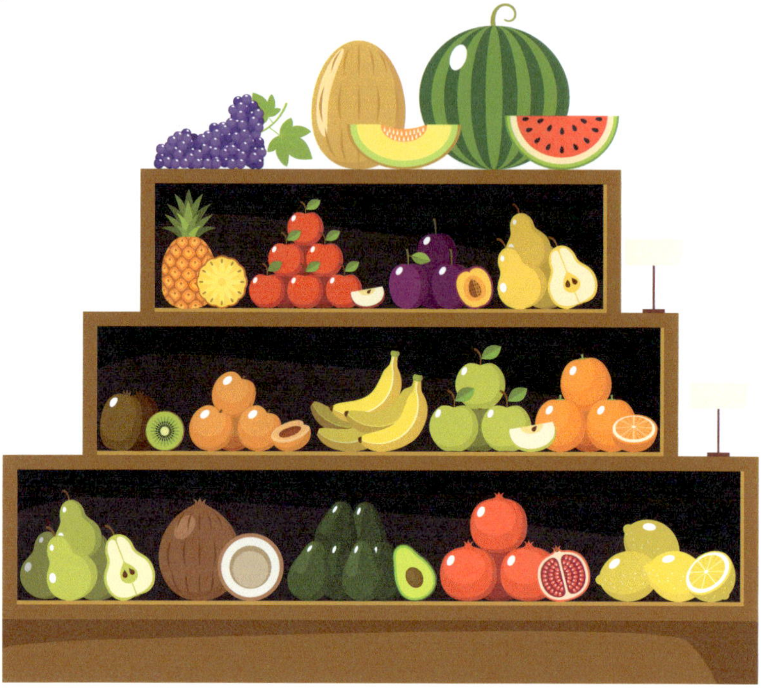

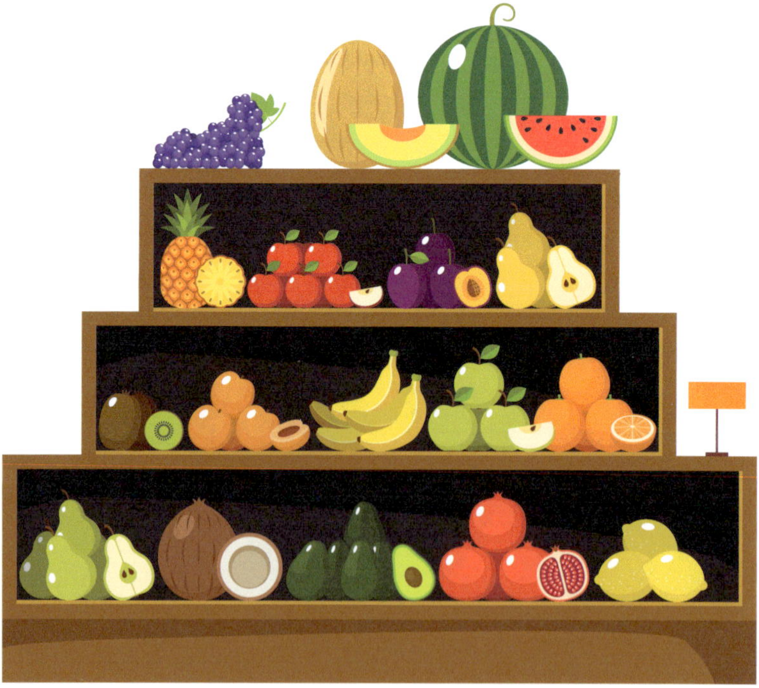

QUIZ TIME

Circle all the Sweet Foods

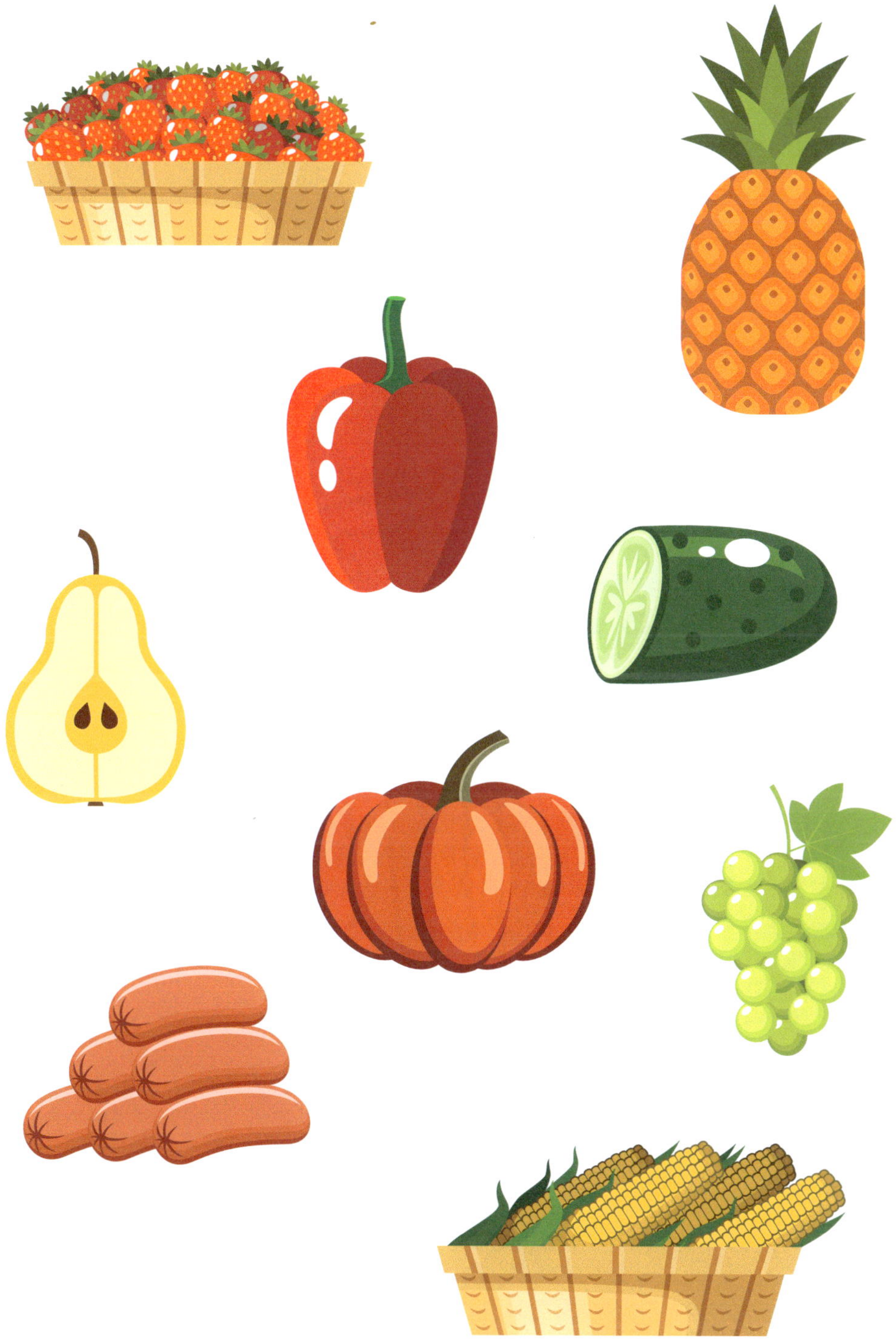

Let's Color

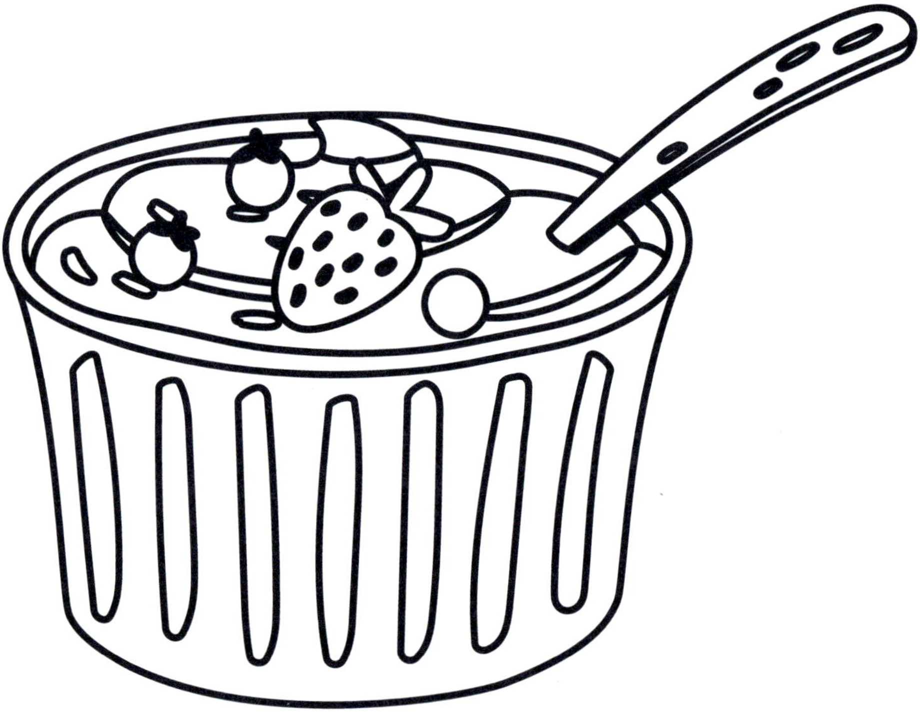

QUIZ TIME

Circle all the Soft Foods

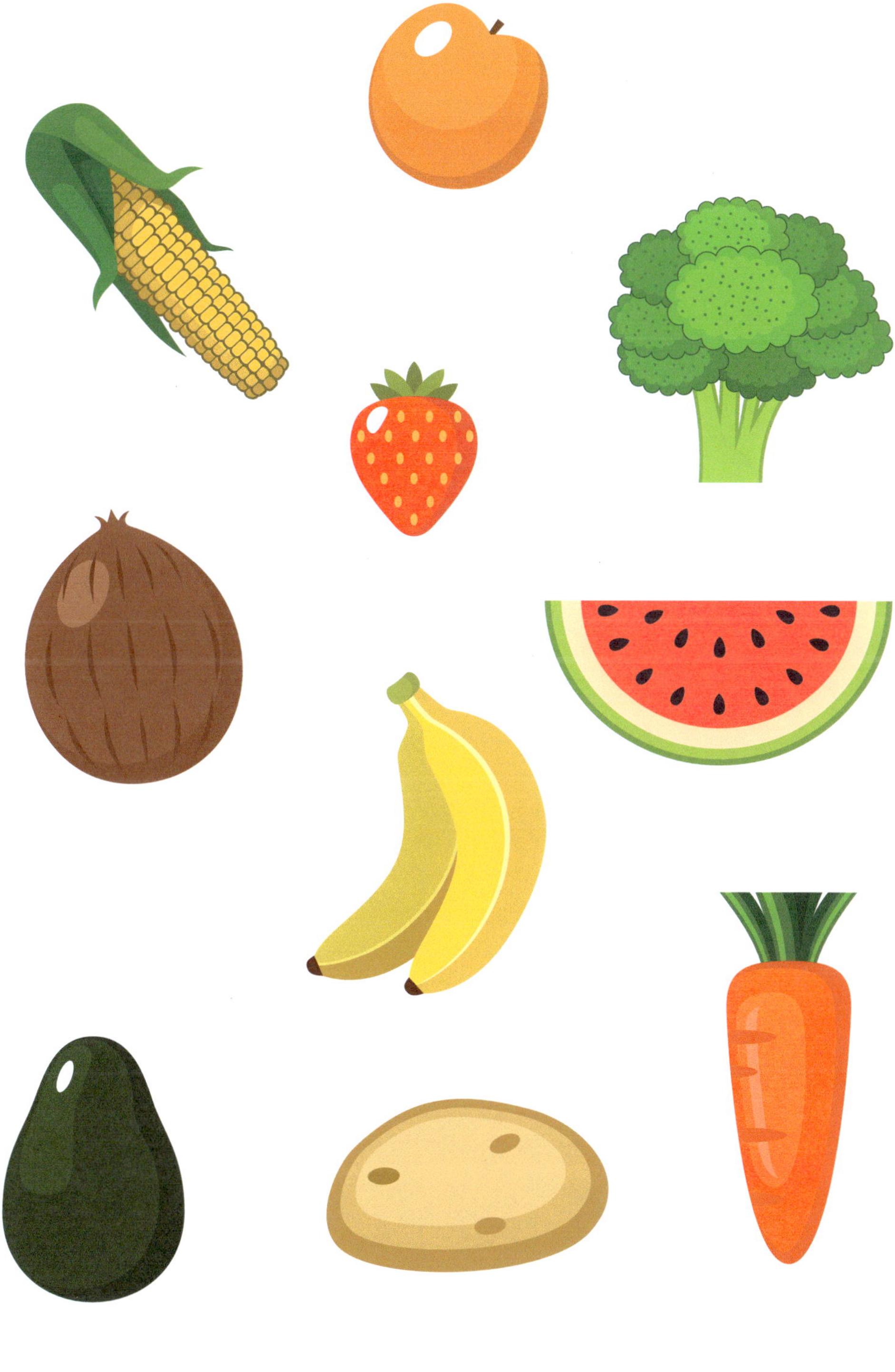

ART TIME

Let's Color

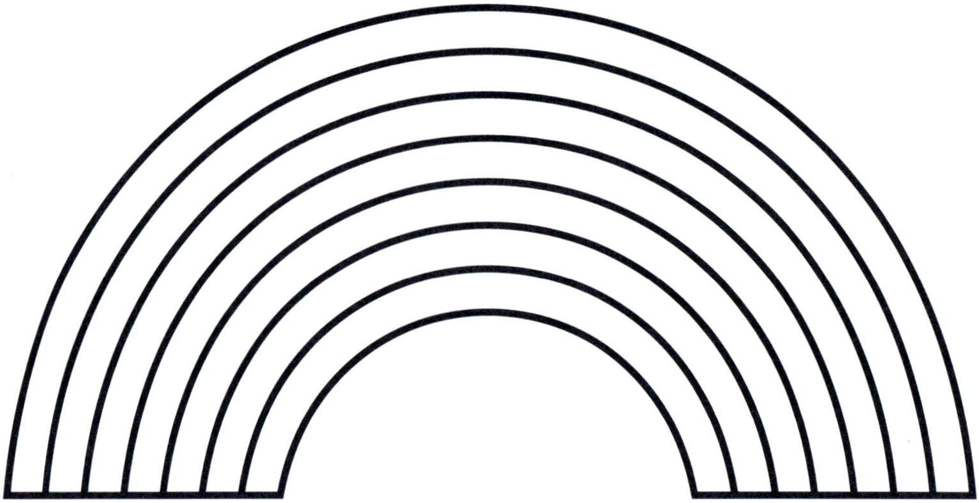

ART TIME

Draw your Favorite Fruit

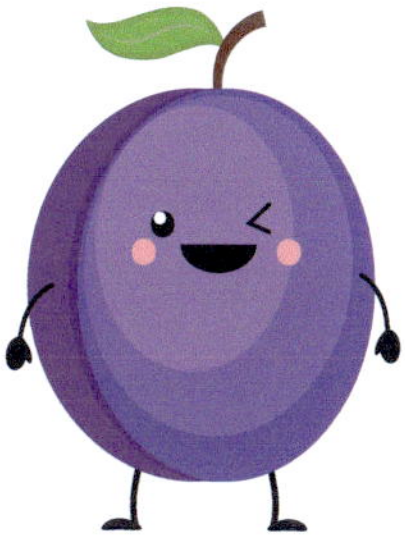

ART TIME

Let's Color

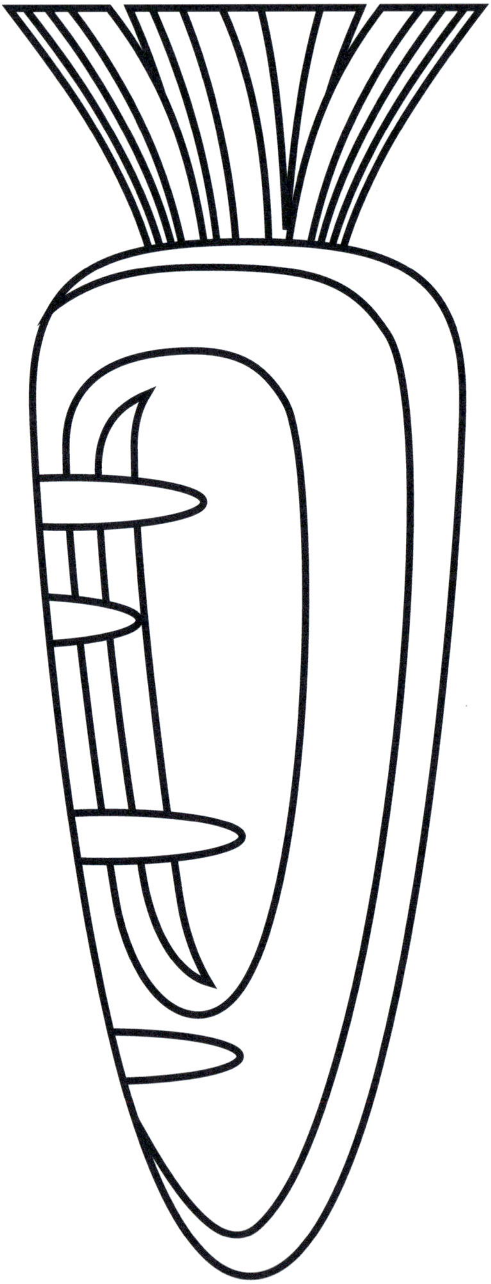

ART TIME

Let's Color

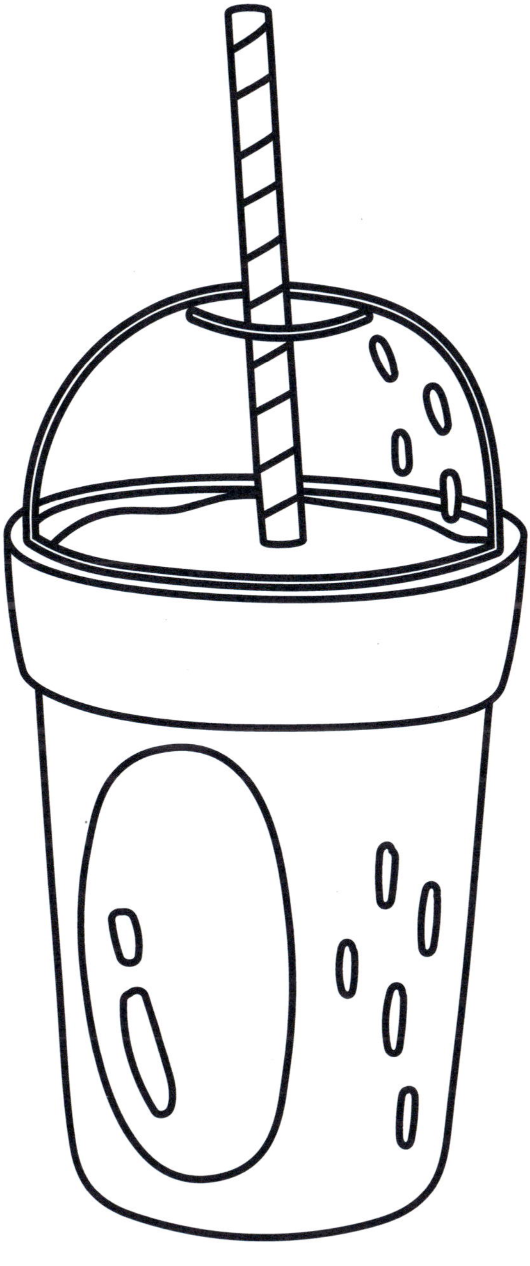

QUIZ TIME

Circle the Foods that would be good in a smoothie

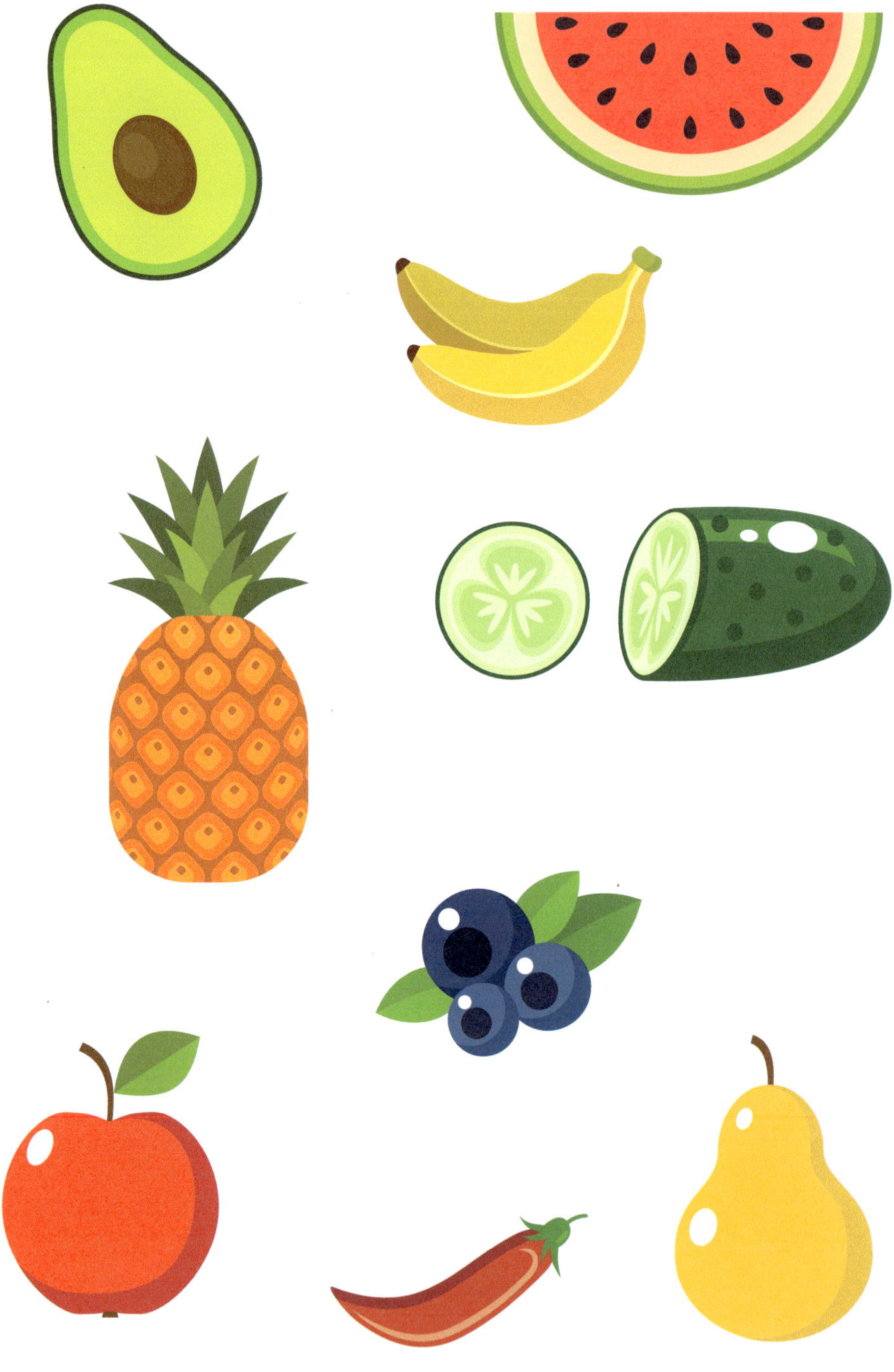

ART TIME

Color and Write your Favorite Fruit

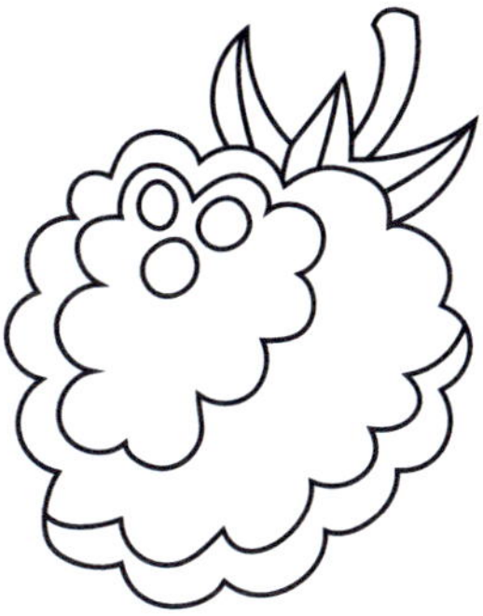

Berries

Melon

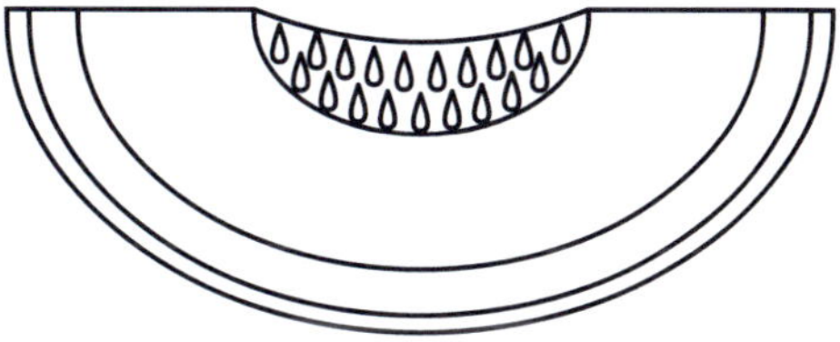

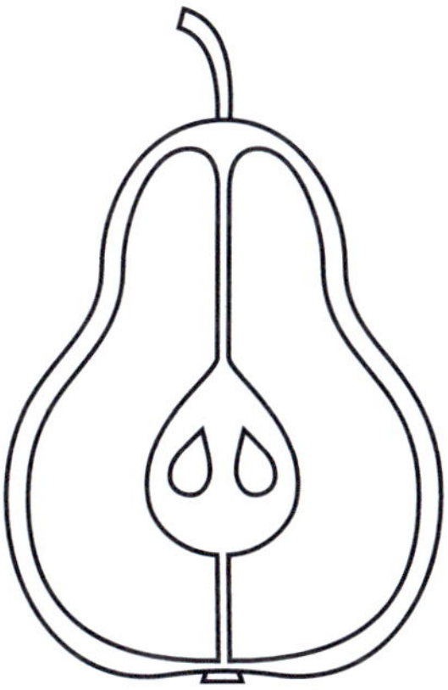

Pear

Apple

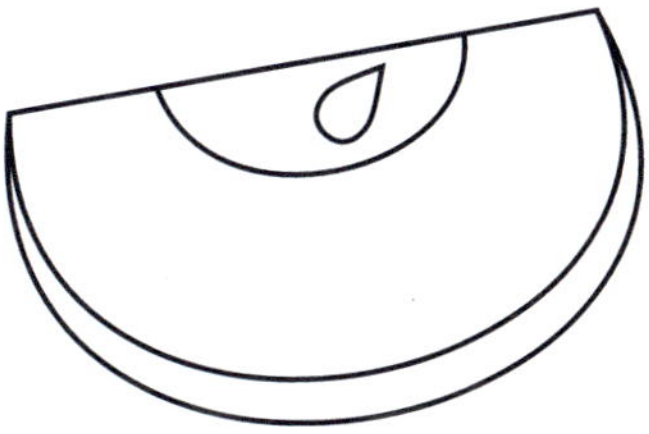

ART TIME

Draw your Favorite Vegetable

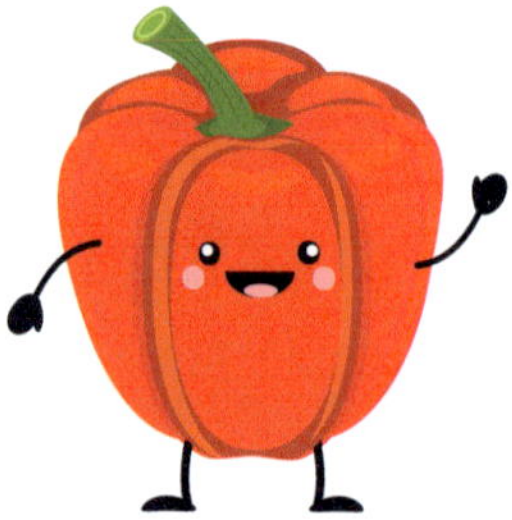

TRIVIA TIME

Circle the Fruits that grow on Trees

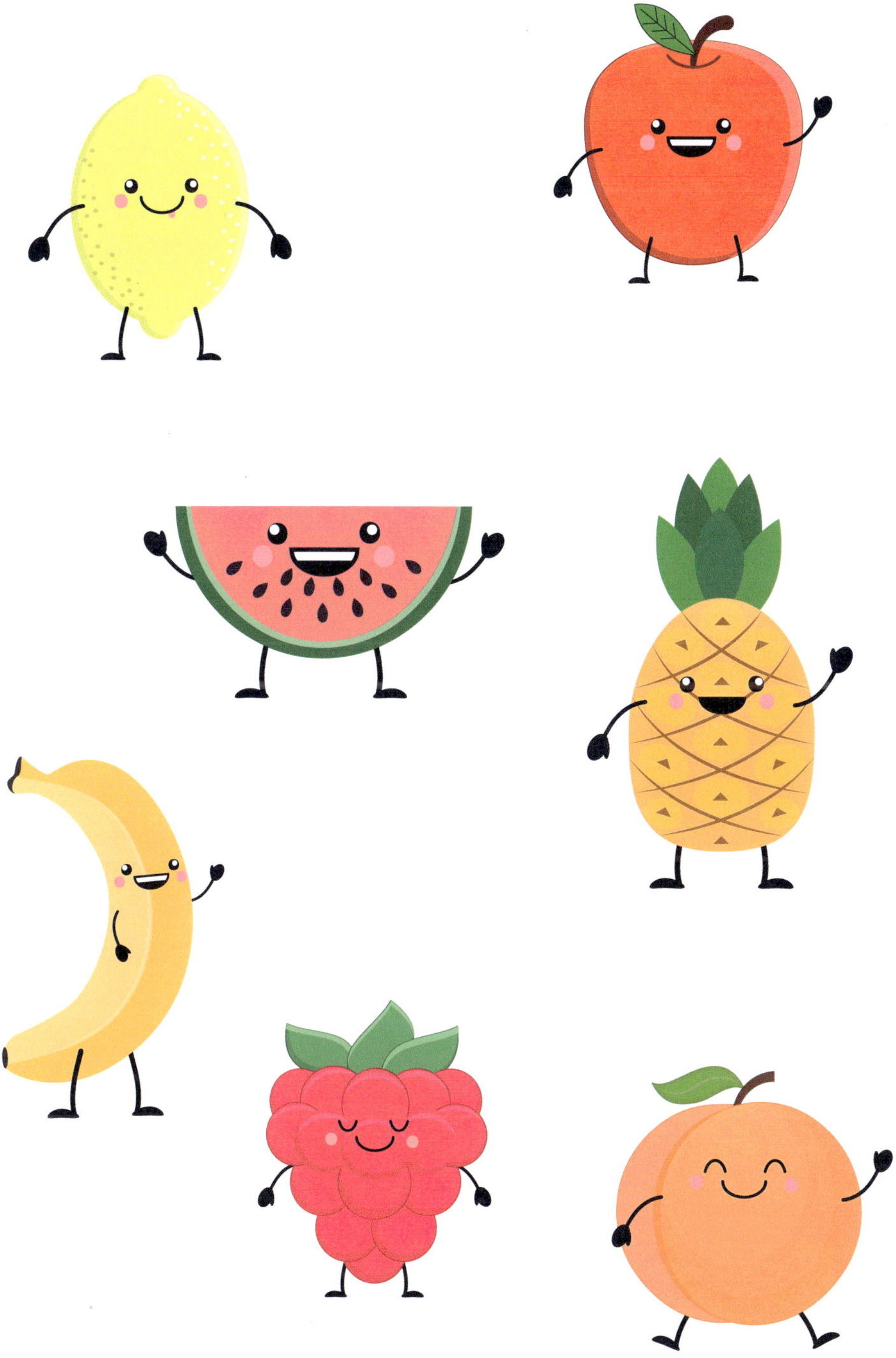

PUZZLE TIME

Find the 10 Differences

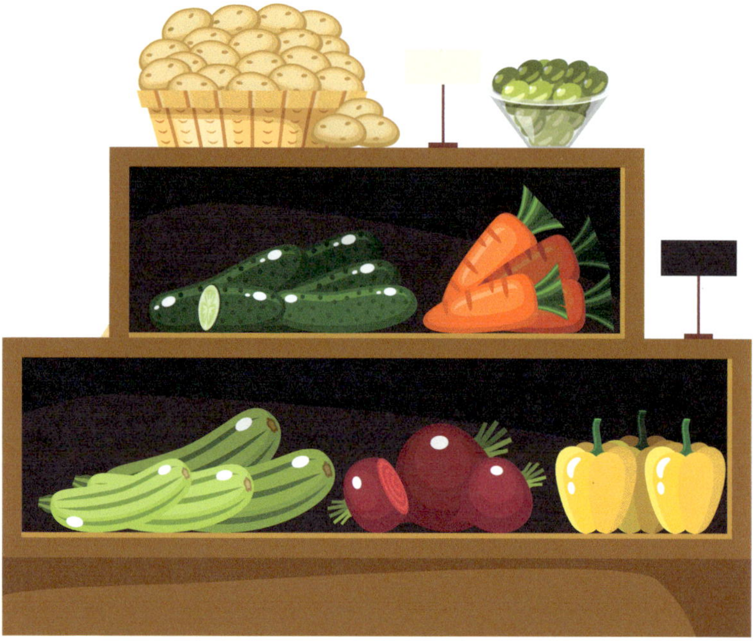

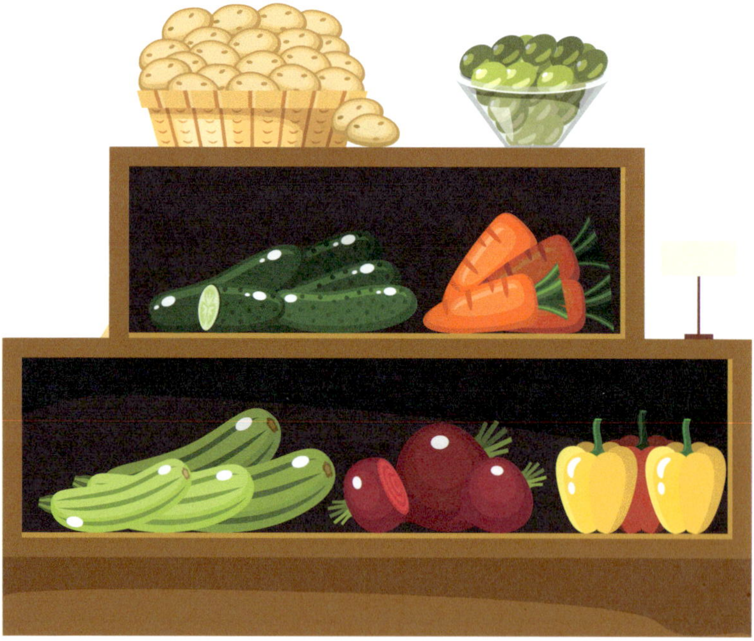

Let's Color

TRIVIA TIME

Find the 5 Differences

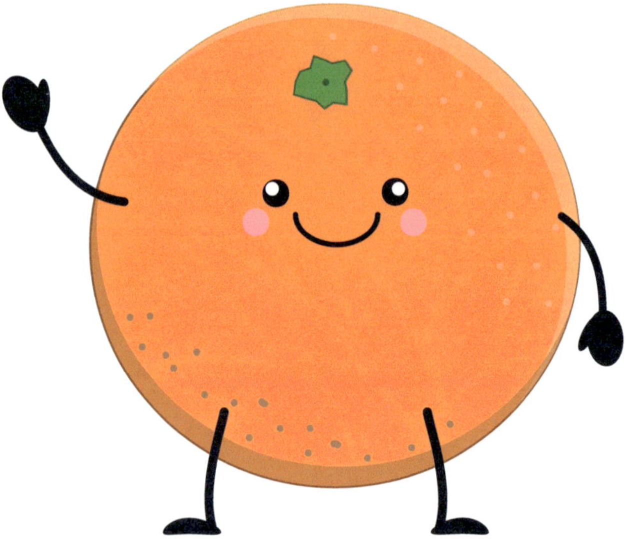

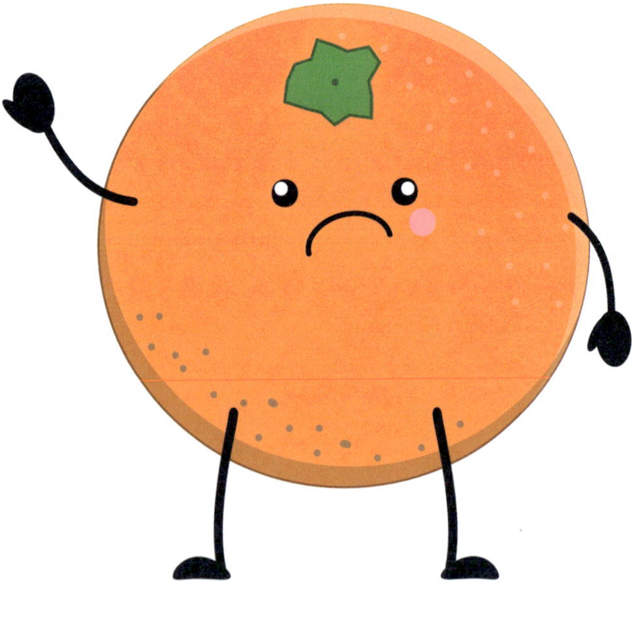

PUZZLE TIME

Color and Write your Favorite Vegetable

Carrot

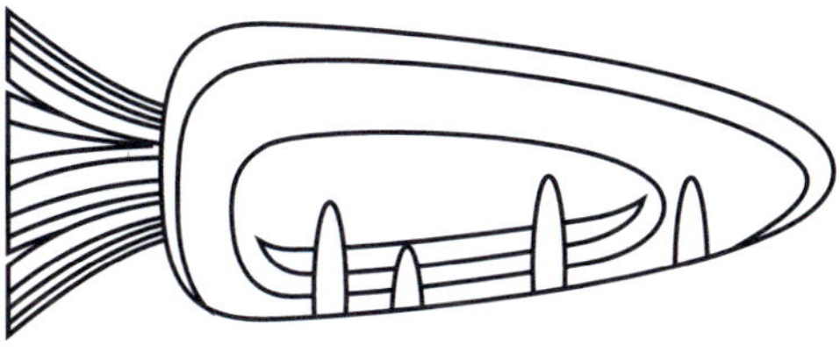

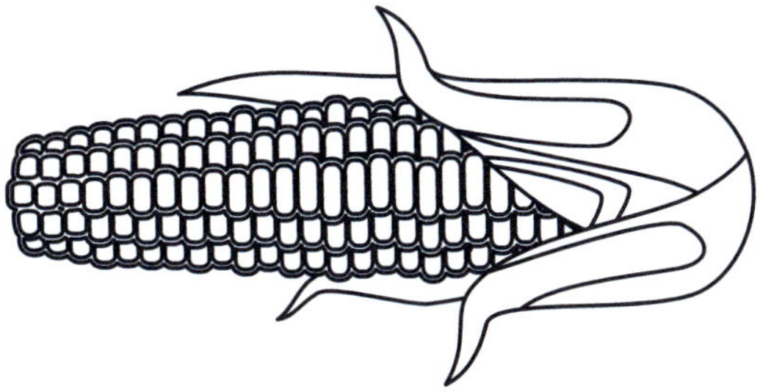

Corn

Cucumber

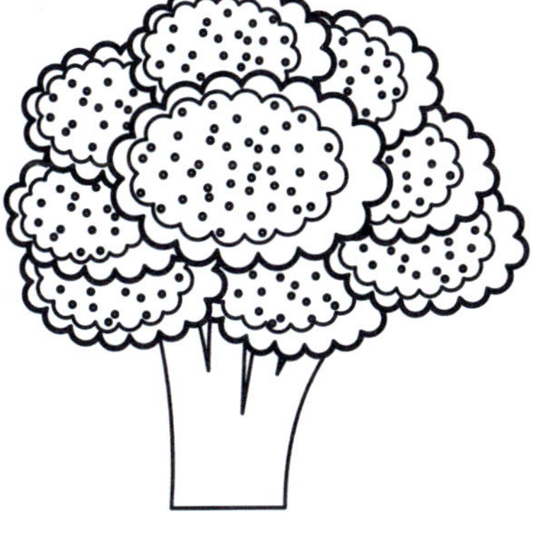

Broccoli

ART TIME

Let's Color

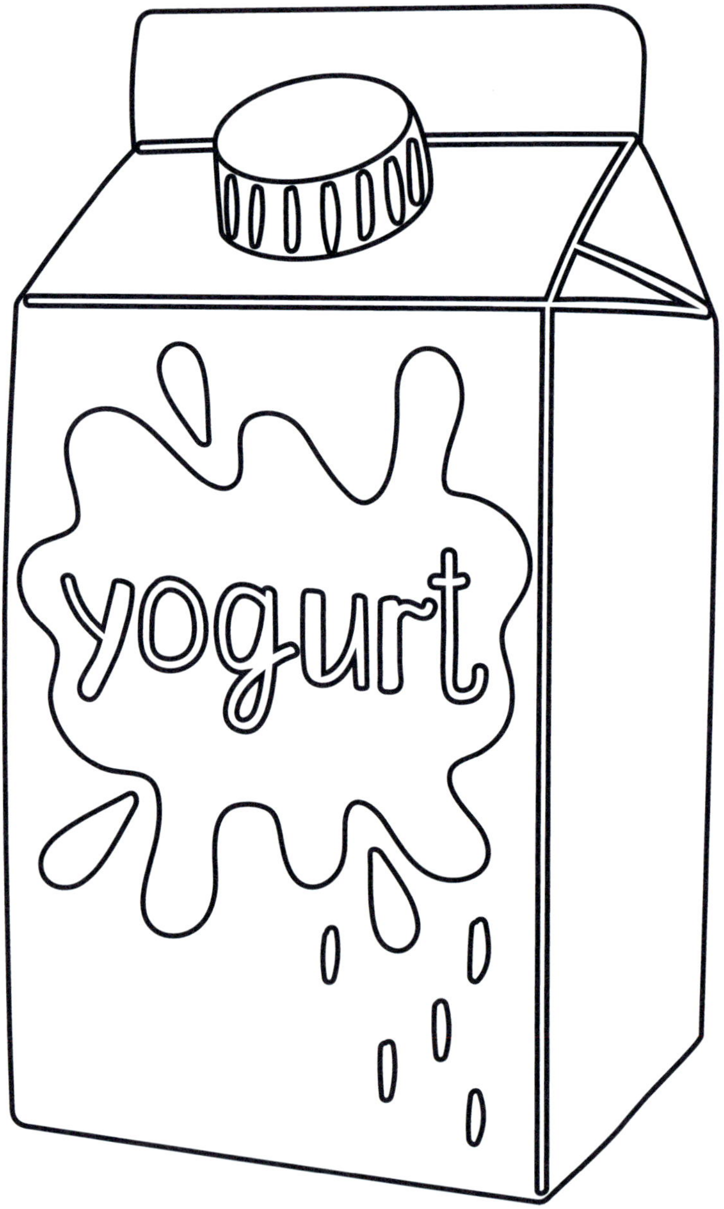

PUZZLE TIME

What Foods do your teeth like?

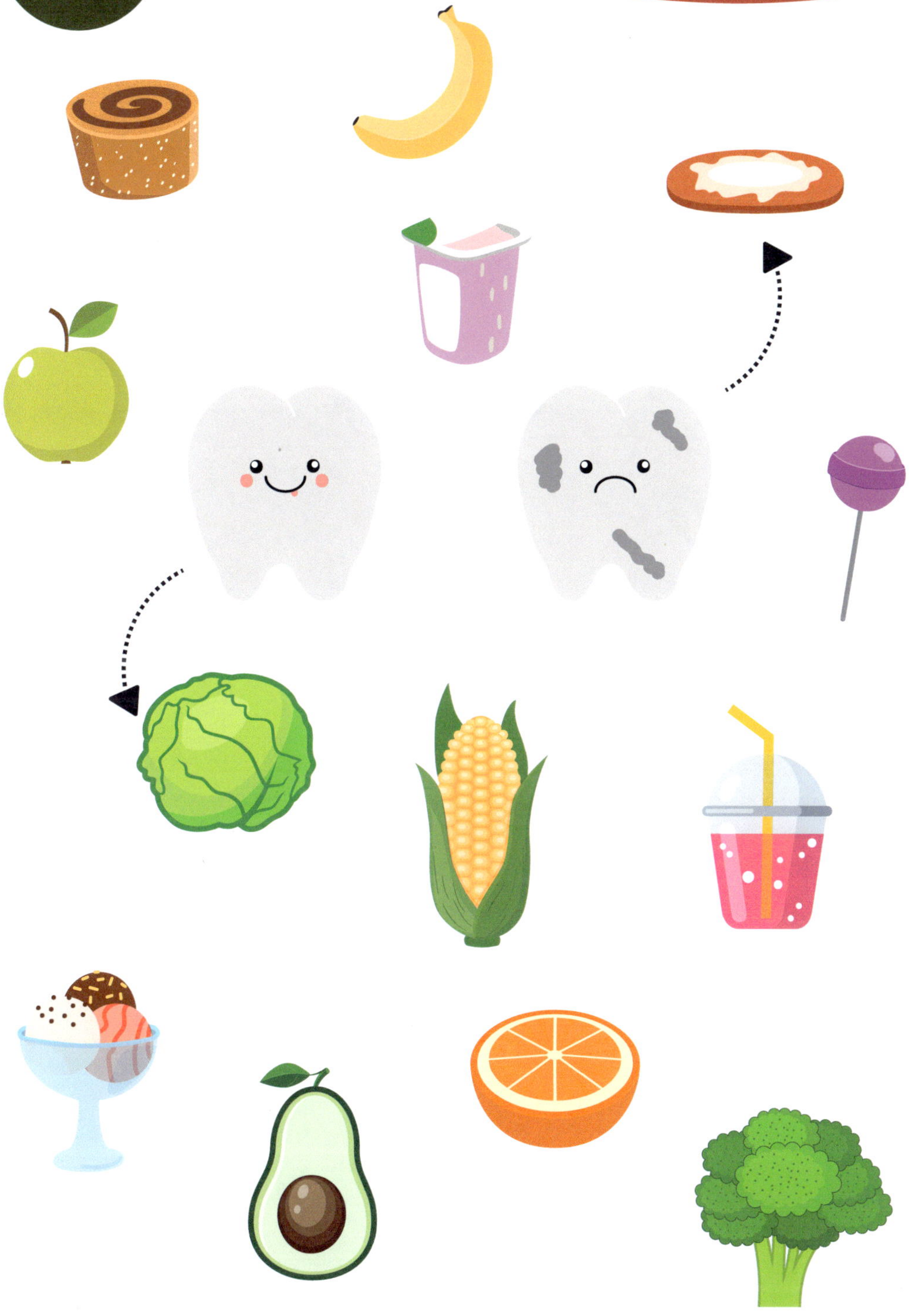

TRIVIA TIME

Circle the Vegetables that grow in the Ground

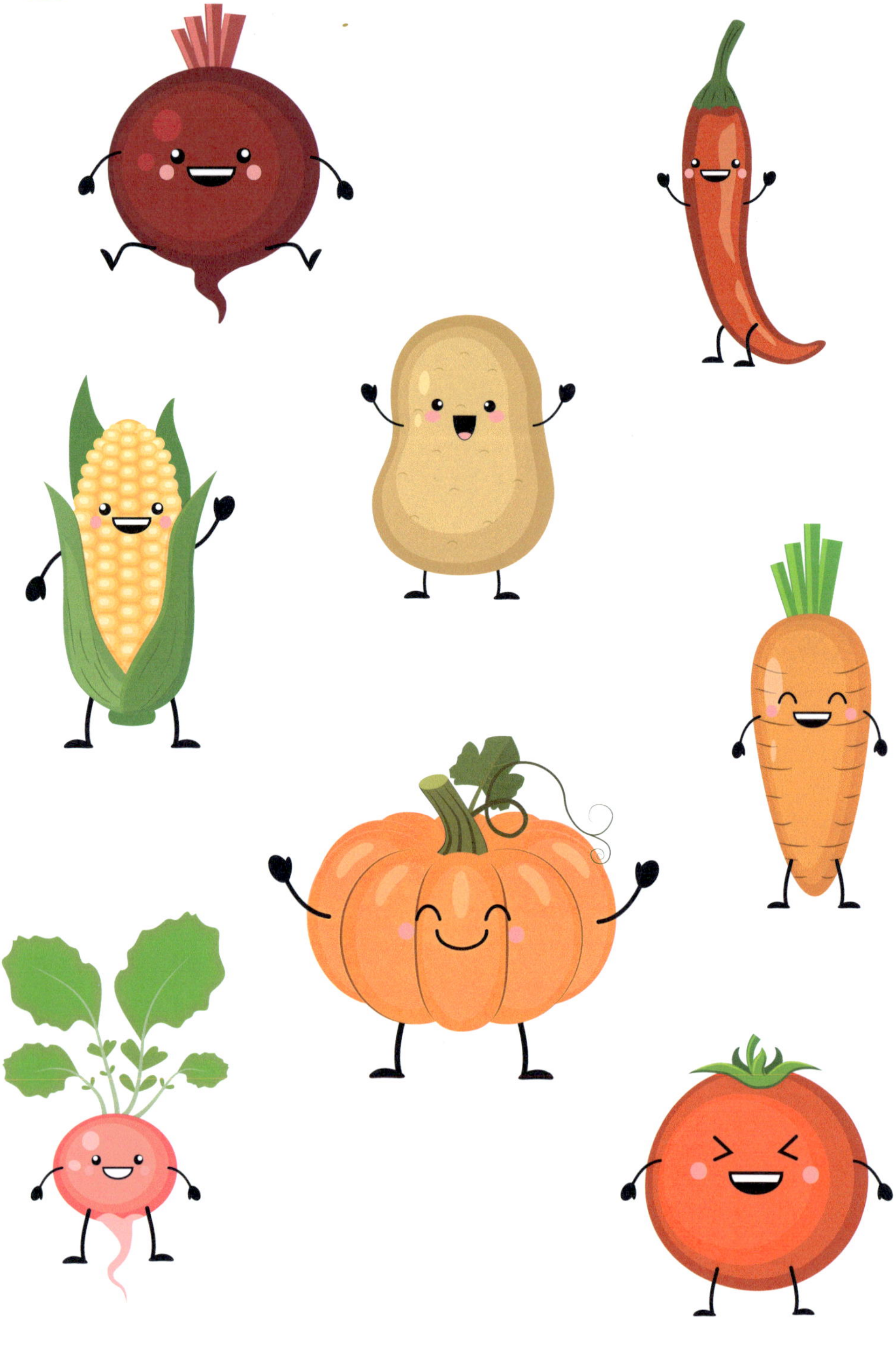

Oven Roasted Cauliflower

Prep Time: 10 minutes • Cook Time: 20 minutes • Total Time: 30 minutes

Ingredients

- 1 medium cauliflower sliced in small florets, or 1/2" thick steaks
- 2 Tbsp olive oil
- 2 Tbsp unsalted butter melted
- ½ tsp garlic powder
- ½ tsp salt or to taste
- ¼ tsp ground paprika
- ¼ tsp ground black pepper or to taste

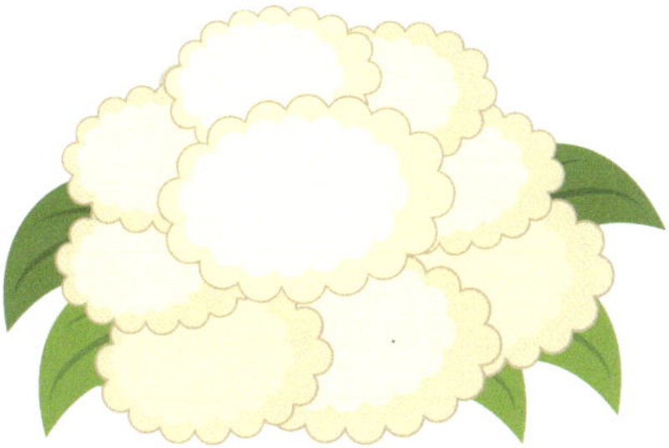

Instructions

1. Preheat the oven to 425°F and line a baking sheet with parchment paper.

2. Slice the head of cauliflower into 1/2" thick steaks, breaking up wedges into even, bite-sized pieces.

3. Add the cauliflower to the center of the baking sheet. Drizzle with the oil and melted butter and toss to combine.

4. In a small bowl, combine garlic powder, salt, paprika, and pepper for the seasoning. Sprinkle onto cauliflower and toss to evenly coat.

5. Spread the cauliflower evenly on the baking sheet and bake at 425°F for 15-20 minutes, until cauliflower reaches desired crispiness.

Recipe Notes

Bake time will slightly vary depending on the side of your florets or slices. You may substitute the butter for oil if you don't want to use any butter.

Baked Parmesan Zucchini

Prep Time: 10 minutes • Cook Time: 20 minutes • Total Time: 30 minutes

Ingredients

- 4 zucchini, quartered lengthwise
- 1/2 cup freshly grated Parmesan
- 1/2 teaspoon dried thyme
- 1/2 teaspoon dried oregano
- 1/2 teaspoon dried basil
- 1/4 teaspoon garlic powder
- Kosher salt and ground black pepper, to taste
- 2 tablespoons olive oil
- 2 tablespoon chopped fresh parsley leaves

Instructions

1. Preheat oven to 350 degrees F. Coat a cooling rack with nonstick spray and place on a baking sheet; set aside.

2. In a small bowl, combine Parmesan, thyme, oregano, basil, garlic powder, salt and pepper, to taste.

3. Place zucchini onto prepared baking sheet. Drizzle with olive oil and sprinkle with Parmesan mixture. Place into oven and bake until tender, about 15 minutes. Then broil for 2-3 minutes, or until crisp and golden brown.

4. Serve immediately, garnished with parsley, if desired.

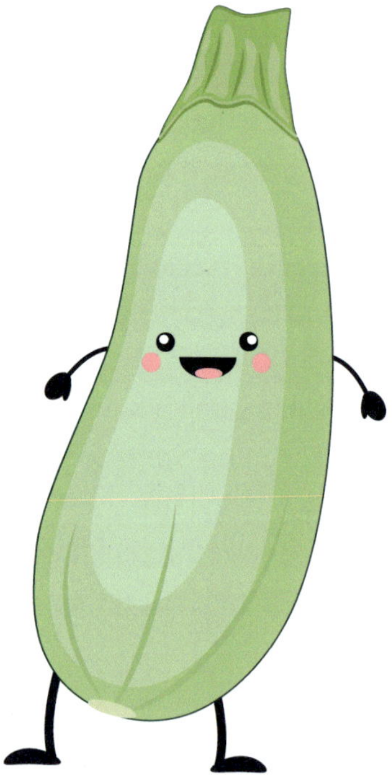

RECIPE TIME

Let's Make Some Food

Baked Beet Chips

Prep Time: 10 minutes • Cook Time: 20 minutes • Total Time: 30 minutes

Ingredients

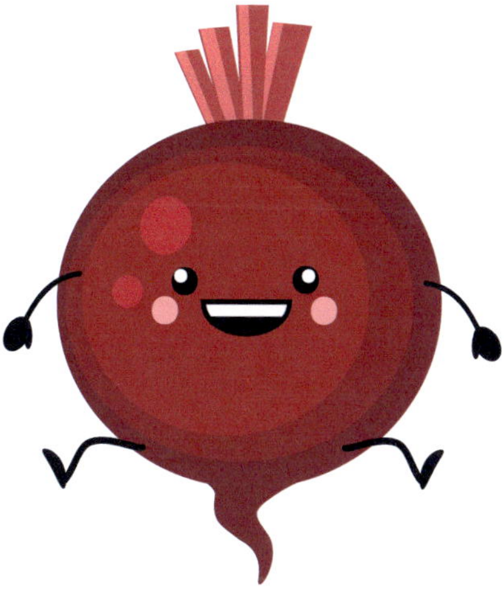

- 6-8 medium to large beets
- Olive oil
- 1 tablespoon flaked sea salt
- 1 tablespoon dried chives

Instructions

1. Trim top and bottom of beets and scrub well under cold water, leaving the skins on. Use a mandoline (or parents could use a sharp knife) to slice the beets 1/16" thin.

2. Preheat the oven to 400° F. Rub small amount of olive oil on baking pan with your hands or a paper towel. (Make sure there is just enough oil so the beets don't stick, but not enough so they cook in the oil or they will steam instead of bake and come out limp instead of crisp). Layer the sliced beets onto the pan being careful not to overlap. Use more than one sheet pan if needed.

3. Bake the chips on the bottom rack of the oven for 10-15 minutes

4. While the beets are baking, pour the salt into a small bowl and crush the dried chives into the salt.

5. Remove from oven and sprinkle with the chive salt. Allow the beets to cool on the pan, they'll crisp as they cool. Once cool, transfer to a cooling rack to continue to dry and crisp.

RECIPE TIME

SUPER Smoothies

Sunny Days

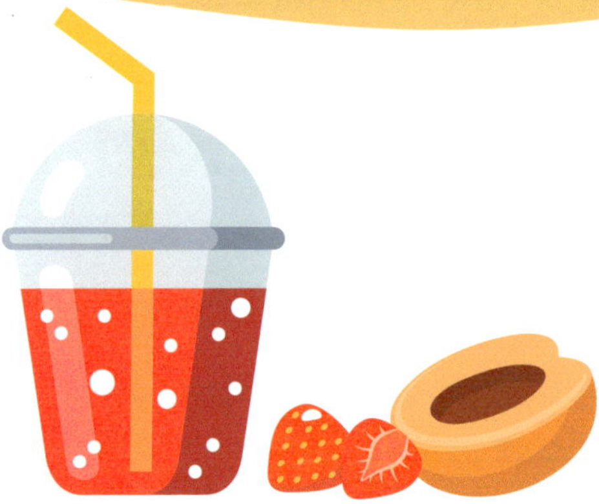

Ingredients

1 cups strawberries

2 peach halves OR 1 bananas

½ cup nonfat plain yogurt

½ cup Almond or Oat milk

Optional

– One envelope instant breakfast mix (for calcium)

– 2 teaspoons honey

– flax seeds or wheat bran

Berry Magic

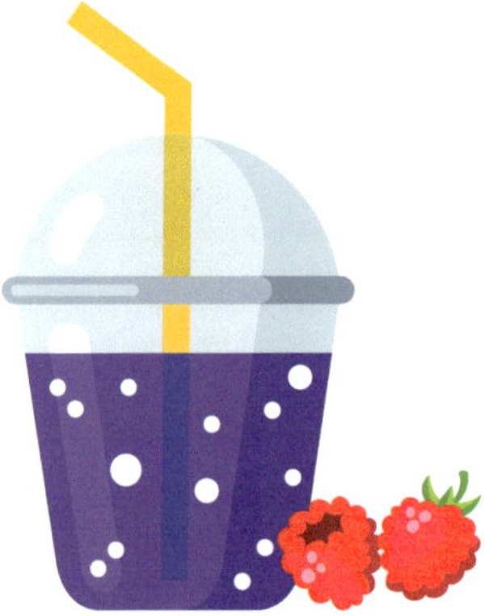

Ingredients

½ cup frozen unsweetened raspberries

½ cup frozen unsweetened blackberries

½ cup nonfat vanilla yogurt

½ cup 2% milk

1 teaspoon vanilla extract

Optional

– pinch cinnamon

– honey

Tropical Waves

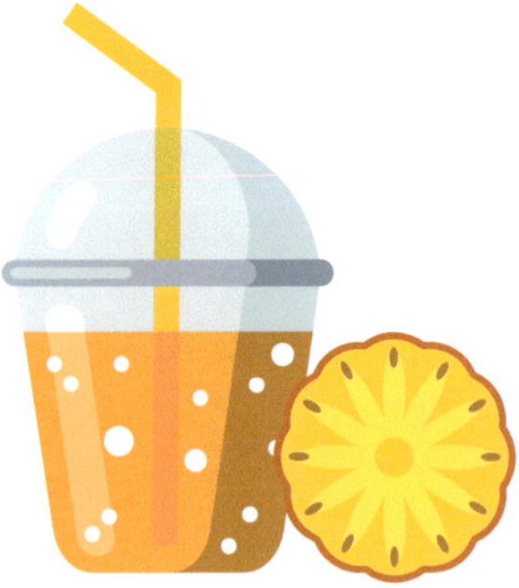

Ingredients

½ cup nonfat plain or vanilla

1 banana sliced

½ cup chopped pineapple

½ orange juice

2 teaspoons vanilla

Ice cubes – OR freeze fruit in advance

RECIPE TIME

SUPER Smoothies

Green Dream

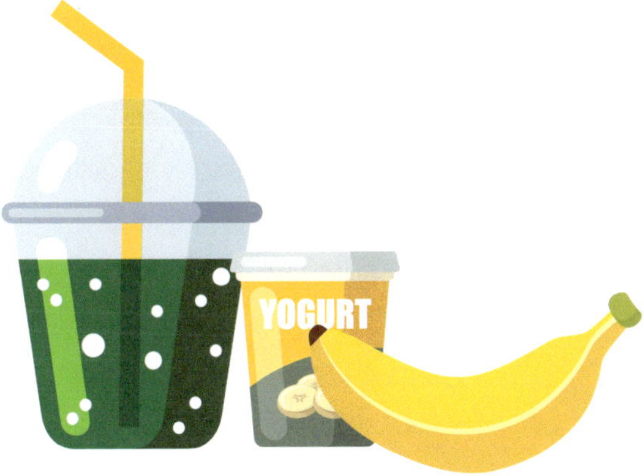

Ingredients

1 cup spinach
1 banana
1 cup nonfat Greek plain yogurt
½ cup Almond milk
1 stalk kale
¼ teaspoon vanilla
Ice cubes

Optional
– 1 scoop protein

Blue Blue Berry

Ingredients

1 cup unsweetened Vanilla Almond milk or water
¾ cup frozen blue berries
¾ cup frozen bananas
¼ cup almond butter

Optional nutrition boosters
– ¼ old fashioned oats
And/or 2 tablespoons flax seeds
– 1 to 2 teaspoons to taste

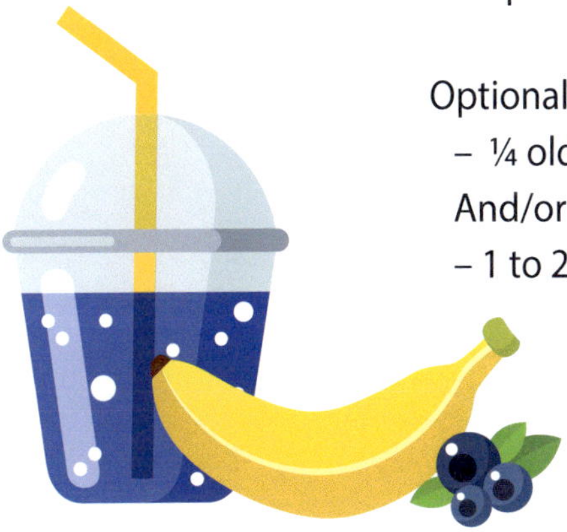

Nutrition

"Nutritionally speaking you are what you eat;
on a cellular level only whole foods complete.
Improper eating always leads to starvation;
whether over- or underweight, it's harsh sensation
prevents you from having energy or thriving.
Lack of nutrients traps you in the mode of just surviving.
Your metabolism determines your level of health;
a great metabolic rate moves you with stealth,
creating the energy output required
so burning fat, exercise, and mental clarity is acquired.
Eating proper nutrients is the master key
that opens the door to being healthy.
There are areas of your body only nutrients can reach;
they protect, flush, or fill and prevent any breach.
Accessing optimal health and changing your current condition
metamorphically happens with a metabolic transition.
The significance of your diet cannot be overstated:
food is actually medicine and can provide the life you've awaited."

Excerpt From: Wendy Falcon. "Turn Your Life Insight Out."

Made in the USA
Monee, IL
05 November 2026

67379322R00036